Plasmapheresis in Immunology and Oncology

Beiträge zur Onkologie
Contributions to Oncology

Vol. 10

Series Editors
S. Eckhardt, Budapest; *J. H. Holzner, Wien, G. A. Nagel,* Göttingen

S. Karger
Basel · München · Paris · London · New York · Tokyo · Sydney

Symposium of Arbeitsgemeinschaft Internistische Onkologie (AIO)
der Deutschen Krebsgesellschaft, Göttingen, December 5–6, 1980

Plasmapheresis in Immunology and Oncology

Volume Editors
J.-H. Beyer, Göttingen; *H. Borberg,* Köln;
Ch. Fuchs und *G. A. Nagel,* Göttingen

101 figures and 44 tables, 1982

S. Karger
Basel · München · Paris · London · New York · Tokyo · Sydney

Beiträge zur Onkologie
Contributions to Oncology

Vol. 8: Nicht-seminomatöse Hodentumoren. AIO-Symposium in Bad Neuenahr, 1981
Herausgeber: H. J. Illiger, Bonn; H. Sack, S. Seeber, Essen; L. Weissbach, Bonn
X + 294 S., 113 Abb., 107 Tab., 1981. ISBN 3-8055-3065-X

Vol. 9: Adriamycin-Symposium. Ergebnisse und Aspekte. Gemeinsames Symposium der Arbeitsgemeinschaft Internistische Onkologie (AIO) der Deutschen Krebsgesellschaft und der Farmitalia Carlo Erba (Freiburg i. Br.) – Frankfurt a. M., 1981
Herausgeber: D. Füllenbach, Freiburg i. Br.; G. A. Nagel, Göttingen; S. Seeber, Essen
X + 462 S., 110 Abb., 5 Farbt., 167 Tab., 1981. ISBN 3-8055-2966-X

National Library of Medicine, Cataloging in Publication

Plasmapheresis in immunology and oncology: symposium of Arbeitsgemeinschaft Internistische Onkologie (AIO) der Deutschen Krebsgesellschaft, Göttingen, December 5–6, 1980 / volume editors, J. H. Beyer . . . [et al.]. – Basel; New York: Karger, 1982.
(Beiträge zur Onkologie; v. 10)
1. Neoplasms – immunology – congresses   2. Neoplasms – therapy – congresses   3. Plasma Exchange – congresses   4. Plasmapheresis – congresses   I. Arbeitsgemeinschaft Internistische Onkologie   II. Beyer, J. H.   III. Series:
Beiträge zur Onkologie; Bd. 10
ISBN 3-8055-3467-1
W1 BE444N Bd. 10
[QZ 200 P715 1980]

Contents

III. Tumor Immune Diagnosis

Chairmen: K. Hoeffken, Essen, and J.-H. Beyer (Göttingen)

IV. Therapeutical Aspects of Plasma Exchange in Cancer Patients

Chairmen: H. Borberg and G. A. Nagel (Göttingen)

Preface

The four main topics of this plasma exchange symposium were:
(1) Technical aspects of different modalities of plasmapheresis and immunoabsorption and their complications,
(2) aspects of general tumor immunology,
(3) tumor immune diagnosis, and
(4) therapeutic aspects of plasma exchange in cancer patients and special immune diseases.

The main goal of this symposium was to answer the following questions:
–   Does the concept of the immunological interaction between tumor and host have to be changed?
–. Which mechanisms are responsible for the failure of the specific or non-specific defense mechanisms of the host?
–   Are serum factors able to influence the course of a tumor?
–   Which diagnostic methods are able to detect these serum factors?
–   Is it possible, reasonable, and justifiable to eliminate these serum factors with plasma exchange or immunoabsorption without enhancing tumors?

In the last few years immunotherapy failed to be effective for cancer patients. In general, it is not necessary to alter the concept that the immunological antitumor reactions are cell mediated. Non-specific serum factors, however, seem to be more important than hitherto expected. The elimination of these factors, e.g. by plasma exchange, seems to be justified if they are able to modulate tumor-defense mechanisms. In vitro assays, especially cell-culture assays, demonstrate the blocking activity of these serum factors. There is little knowledge about the nature of such factors. Furthermore, the biological relevance of these factors in the individual course of a patient's disease is also still unknown.

Few clinical studies suggest that the elimination of serum-blocking substances are of prognostic value for tumor patients. Circulating immune complexes are of main interest. Their identification and characterization may help to establish monoclonal antitumor antibodies and thereafter to eliminate these factors by tumorspecific immunoabsorption.

In a number of cancer patients it was possible to overcome drug resistance by eliminating the serum-blocking factors.

Tumor enhancement could not be demonstrated in any cancer patient.

Plasmapheresis, e.g. performed by blood-cell separators, membrane filtration, or other techniques, and immunoabsorption are still experimental procedures for cancer patients. The first experiences of groups in Sweden, France, USA, and Germany seem to justify the continuation of this work under strict observation of clinical conditions.

Further work has to be done in developing new techniques: e.g. new membranes, new and more specific immunoabsorbants, filtration procedures; and in researching the nature of the immunosuppressive factors.

I want to thank the Senate Commission for Cancer Research of the Deutsche Forschungsgemeinschaft in the Ministry for Youth, Family, and Health, as well as Behringwerke/Marburg, Braun/Melsungen, Diamed/Cologne, IBM/Munich, and Travenol/Munich for their financial support.

J.-H. Beyer

I. Technical Aspects of Plasmapheresis and Complications

Chairmen:
Ch. Fuchs and *K. W. Rumpf,* Göttingen

Membrane-Plasma Filtration

*H. J. Gurland[1], Y. Nosé[2], Y. Asanuma[2], M. Blumenstein[1],
P. S. Malchesky[2], W. Samtleben[1], B. Schmidt[1], I. Zawicki[2]*

[1] Med. Klinik I, Klinikum Großhadern, Universität München, FRG
[2] Dept. of Artificial Organs, Cleveland Clinic Foundation, Cleveland Clinic, Ohio, USA

Separation of plasma from whole blood for treatment of various disease states has experienced an increasing number of applications during recent years. Especially in immunologically mediated diseases, immunosuppressive medication is frequently reinforced by plasmaphereses. For a decade now plasma separation has been performed by centrifuges which have undergone considerable technical improvements in recent years.

Through the increased understanding of plasma exchange and its various possibilities a new continuous extracorporeal process has emerged which permits separation of plasma from whole blood by highly porous membranes. Membrane-plasma separation is a relatively simple procedure and can be performed in any institution where there is experience with extracorporeal circulation. This might be the reason why membrane-plasma separation has found its way into many nephrology units – and also because of the present trend to treat immunological diseases of the kidney by plasma exchange. It has to be taken into consideration, however, that plasma filtration differs considerably in some essential aspects from dialysis or hemofiltration.

Since April 1979 we have performed more than 170 membrane-plasma separations in 36 patients using the Plasmaflo® hollow-fiber filter (Asahi Medical Inc., Tokyo). The membrane consists of cellulose-di-acetate with a wall thickness of 160 μ, an inside diameter of 370 μ and a maximum pore diameter of 0.2 μ. The effective surface area of the filter is 0.65 m².

The plasma separations were conducted by arterio-venous or veno-

venous pathways, corresponding to conventional hemodialysis access. At a blood-flow rate of 100 ml/min, about 30 ml plasma/min can be separated. For an individual treatment lasting about 90 min, the average amount of heparin needed for anticoagulation was 7,000 u. The exchange volume was usually in the range of 2–3 l/session. Human albumin diluted to 2.5 % in an electrolyte solution was found to be the most satisfactory replacement fluid.

We have observed that the transport properties of the filter deteriorate during the course of the treatment. These changes, which can be minimized by a proper selection of operating conditions, are caused by:
(a) entrapment and sorption of macromolecules within the membrane pores;
(b) the deposition of formed blood elements at the surface of the membrane as a result of the drag force created by filtration; and
(c) clotting mechanisms.

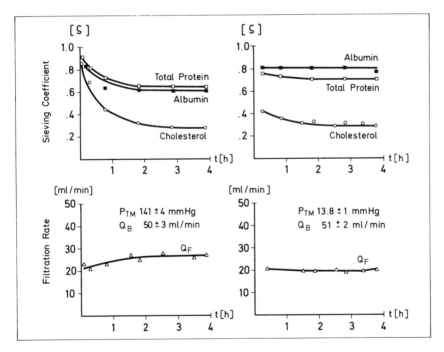

Fig. 1. In vitro test demonstrating change in sieving coefficients and filtrate flow with time at high (left hand) and low (right hand) transmembrane pressure.

Thus, the filtration coefficient as well as the sieving coefficient for proteins will change during the course of the treatment. Since in part these changes are irreversible, membrane modules for plasma separation can hardly be reused.

Due to the high complexity of plasma separation, no complete mathematical theory yet exists to describe the process. The principal factors influencing the technique and experimental quantitative data were published in detail elsewhere [4]. We will discuss only a few parameters here and have chosen those which are most relevant for selection of optimal operating conditions in the clinical application.

Figure 1 illustrates the relationship between transmembrane pressure, filtration rate, and sieving coefficients. As TMP decreases by one order of magnitude, from 141–14 mmHg, the filtration rate decreases by approximately 25%. At the higher transmembrane pressure, the sieving coefficients for proteins decrease within 1 h from initial 0.9 to 0.7, and for the final 2 h of the 4-h test they are in the range of 0.6. In contrast, at the lower TMP, the sieving coefficient for albumin and for total protein is greater than 0.8 and is more stable over the whole period of the experiment. Thus, at the lower TMP, the decrease in filtration rate is compensated to a large degree by the increase of the sieving coefficient. Therefore the lower operating pressures are recommended.

Blood properties, such as hematocrit, platelet count, protein and cholesterol concentration, seem to be the most important factors influencing permeability in plasma separation if one assumes that the amount of heparin used is sufficient to prevent clotting. Among the proteins, cryo-proteins, immune complexes, and immunologically active proteins will make the greatest contribution in changing membrane properties. Proportions of the mentioned blood constituents are related to disease state. Therefore, indirectly, the plasma-separation process is quite dependent on the clinical situation of a patient treated with plasmapheresis.

Figure 2, in which the TMP required to achieve a constant filtration rate is plotted, illustrates the role plasma components play in filtration. The concentration of platelets, which may be considered responsible for the transmembrane pressure, is normal but the total cholesterol level is very high in a patient with primary biliary cirrhosis. On the other hand, platelet count is very high and the total cholesterol level is low in another patient suffering from rheumatoid arthritis. These data suggest that the cholesterol concentration plays by far a larger role in the mechanism of filtration than does the platelet count.

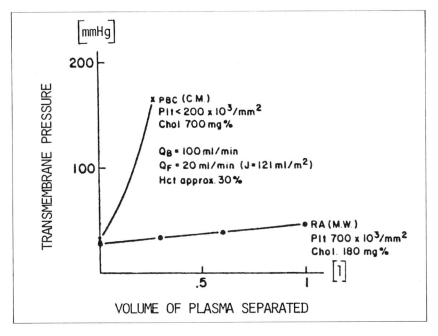

Fig. 2. Comparison of transmembrane-pressure data for patients with primary biliary cirrhosis (PBC) and rheumatoid arthritis (RA).

Another example for the relationship between disease state and plasma separation is demonstrated in figure 3 where the transmembrane pressure is given vs. the volume of plasma treated in 4 consecutive treatments of the same rheumatoid-arthritis patient in 1-week intervals. This decrease of the minimum required transmembrane pressure in the course of 4 consecutive treatments is consistent with a steady decrease of the immune complex concentration determined by C_{1q}-binding.

It is important to draw attention to the fact that, when combining different types of membranes and technologies, a selective removal of offending proteins will be possible in the future. One of the potential protocols is the so-called double-filtration plasmapheresis which is dealt with in this symposium. Since cryoglobulins are present in various diseases of the immune system, the authors in Cleveland [2] and in Munich have been gathering clinical experiences with on-line macromolecule separation and consecutive cryogelation. In this specific mode of selective plasma separation, plasma is at first separated on-line from whole blood using a membrane hollow-fiber filter whose sieving properties for plasma

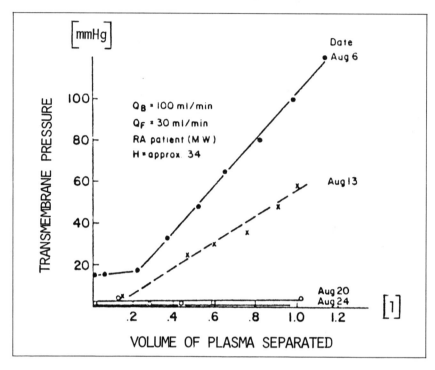

Fig. 3. Consecutive treatments in patient with rheumatoid arthritis, demonstrating a decrease of transmembrane pressure with consecutive treatments.

proteins are approximately 100%. The separated plasma is then cooled to 4°C and directed to a second membrane filter that retains plasma proteins greater than the size of albumin, while passing plasma solutes the size of albumin or less. The cooling improves the removal of plasma proteins that cryogelate or cryoprecipitate. The filtered plasma is then united with the mainstream blood flow which is warmed before being returned to the patient. Since the purified plasma is given back to the patient on-line, there is minimal requirement for the infusion of plasma products.

In an earlier publication [3], we showed that immunoglobulin levels can be significantly reduced to about 60% of their initial values. Likewise, the concentration of one of the mediators of the inflammatory process – fibrinogen – is usually reduced to about 50% but gradually rebounds within the next 24 to 48 hrs without, however, reaching its initial value.

Although enthusiastic about the fact that we are able to eliminate pathogenetic proteins, we nevertheless have to ask ourselves what other substances are simultaneously eliminated during a non-selective plasma exchange.

In a 2 l plasma exchange with the Plasmaflo® and the substitution fluid employed by us, electrolytes and albumin remain in balance but the total protein concentration decreases by about 20% (fig. 4).

Likewise, the levels of urea, creatinine, uric acid, and phosphate remain nearly unchanged. On the other hand, cholesterol and triglycerides are reduced to about 50% of their pre-treatment levels (fig. 5).

The concentration of the 5 enzymes shown in figure 6 is lowered by about 30% during a 2 l plasma exchange. Clinical experience teaches us that this reduction of pre-treatment values does not cause any side effects. Normalization which is usually reached within a few hours – with the exception of serum lipis – depends upon initial concentration, compartment distribution within the body, and the generation rate.

In this context, changes of cellular blood components should also be emphasized. The filtration process will necessarily increase the hematocrit but the outlet value for the hematocrit should not exceed 65% in order to prevent blood-cell damage and particle deposition on the membrane.

Leucocyte behavior shows a marked decrease of white cells after 20 min for the Plasmaflo® separator (fig. 7). This phenomenon is non-specific

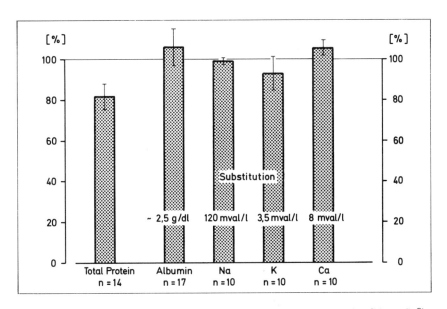

Fig. 4. Deviation of initial value after 2 l of membrane plasma separation (Plasmaflo®).

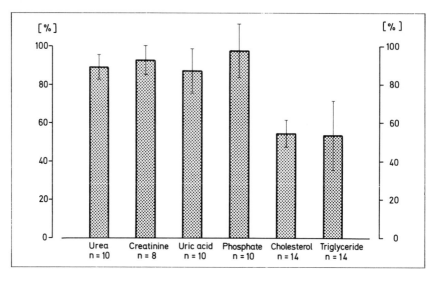

Fig. 5. Deviation of initial value after 2 l of membrane plasma separation (Plasmaflo®).

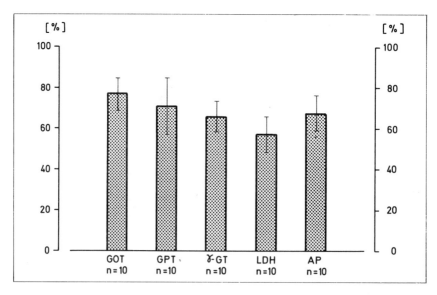

Fig. 6. Deviation of initial value after 2 l of membrane plasma separation (Plasmaflo®).

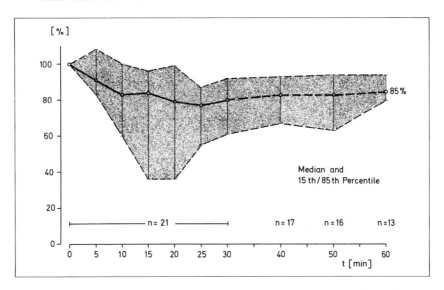

Fig. 7. Leukocyte response to membrane-plasma separation (Plasmaflo®). Median and 15th/85th percentile.

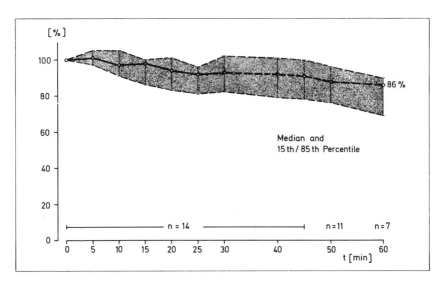

Fig. 8. Platelet response to membrane-plasma separation (Plasmaflo®). Median and 15th/85th percentile.

and similar to that noted using cellulosic membranes in various extracorporeal treatment schemes [1].

A similar decrease of 14% occurs in platelet count after 1 h although here the deviation is considerably less (fig. 8). These data indicate that platelet activation or damage might occur. However, this decrease is less dramatic than the platelet loss of 30% per treatment observed with centrifugal techniques.

In conclusion:
(1) Plasma filtration differs from dialysis techniques by the type of membranes used and their tendency to change properties during the process.
(2) Membrane-plasma filtration offers possibilites for a selective separation of pathogenetic substances.
(3) The concentration of macromolecules can be reduced up to 50% per exchange.
(4) No obvious side effects were observed as a result of a temporary reduction in serum enzymes and blood-count changes.
(5) Membrane-plasma separation now can be considered a safe and clinically applicable mode of treatment.

References

1   Jacob, A. I.; Gavellas, G.; Zarco, R.; Perez, G.; Bourgoignie, J. J.: Leukopenia, hypoxia, and complement function with different hemodialysis membranes. Kidney int. *18:* 505–509 (1980).
2   Malchesky, P. S.; Asanuma, Y.; Zawicki, I.; Blumenstein, M.; Calabrese, L.; Kyo, A.; Krakauer, R.; Nosé, Y: On-line separation of macromolecules by membrane filtration with cryogelation. Artificial Organs *4:* 205–207 (1980).
3   Samtleben, W.; Blumenstein, M.; Liebl, L.; Gurland, H. J.: Membrane-plasma separation for treatment of immunologically mediated diseases. Trans. Am. Soc. artif. internal Organs *26:* 12–16 (1980).
4   Zawicki, I.; Malchesky, P. S.; Asanuma, Y.; Smith, J. W.; Kyo, A.; Blumenstein, M.; Shinagawa, S.; Kayashima, K.; Nosé, Y.: Quantitation of membrane-plasma filtration. Presented at ISAO/IFAC Symposium on Control Aspects of Artificial Organs, September 24–26, 1980, Warsaw/Poland (in press, 1981).

Prof. Dr. med. Hans J. Gurland, Leiter der Nephrolog. Abt., Medizin. Klinik I, Klinikum Großhadern der Universität München, Marchioninistr. 15, D-8000 München 70

Technical Aspects of Cell-Plasma Separation and the Elimination of Plasma-Components ex Vivo

Helmut Borberg

Medizinische Universitätsklinik, Labor für Tumorimmunologie, Köln, FRG

The elimination of protein-bound pathogenic material, though of interest for the treatment of many diseases, has rarely been used or taken into consideration for many years until 1969. This nowadays surprising phenomenon may be explained with the lack of an appropriate technology. However, conventional centrifugation, using the double bag technique for the separation and removal of plasma from cells, has long been available prior to the introduction of the more fashionable techniques [1]. As an inexpensive and effective tool of therapy, it is still the method of choice at those places where plasma exchange is not in regular use, provided that a proper handling and organization can be set up.

Since 1969 when blood-cell separators were first used for plasma exchange [3, 5], this improvement of the centrifugation of blood components developed to a most elegant, effective and, when compared to other technologies, inexpensive method. It is now used in approximately more than 90 % of all therapeutic plasmapheresis procedures. Continuous and intermittent flow systems are available and compete with each other. Each has its advantages and disadvantages.

Continuous flow systems are represented by the IBM/NIH model 2990 and the Aminco Celltrifuge, which were the first machines available for routine use, and by the IBM model 2997 and the Aminco Celltrifuge II, which represent the improved technology.

The discontinuous or intermittent flow system originally derive from the Cohn fractionator and are mainly represented by the Haemonetics Model 30 and recently also by the Bellco Progress. The Haemonetics

PEX-system and the Travenol CS 3000 are recent models, characterized by full automatization.

The continuous-flow principle offers the advantage of procedural briefness as compared to the discontinuous systems, if a twofold access to the circulation can be accomplished. Alternatively, the discontinuous systems need more time for the exchange procedure because of the retransfusion of the extracorporeal fluid. The disadvantage has been considerably reduced in the new Haemonetics PEX-system, which accelerates the return flow by using a pump instead of gravity. Also it is the first fully automated system available. The most outstanding advantage of the discontinuous flow systems is that plasma-exchange therapy can be performed with a single needle.

Technical equipment, which allows each variable of the operation to be influenced separately, is now available for all types of centrifugal systems, whereas older models lack this kind of flexibility. Convenient mobility, an advantage over the discontinuous systems, is not decisive but may be of considerable help for certain clinical conditions, if, for instance, supported respiration requires that the machine be moved rather than the patient.

The length of the procedure – and this refers also to other than centrifugal techniques – is defined by the flow rate rather than the technique of cell-plasma separation (table I). The flow rate depends on the type of access to the patient's circulation and this again depends on the patient's venous system. Plasma-exchange therapy can generally be performed either on a veno-venous or a single venous flow basis. Thus an artificial access to the circulation using catheters, fistulae or shunts bearing rare but serious side effects is generally unacceptable, except for emergencies or patients with inaccessible cubital veins. Since blood-cell separators have a wide range of continuously adjustable pump rates ranging from 20–100 ml/min and more, they can also be operated using a central venous or arterio-venous access, if this cannot be avoided.

The anticoagulation can be performed with both heparin or citrate. The volume of the applied anticoagulant contributes to the hemodilution, limiting the efficacy of the plasma exchange. Since heparin is generally applied in a more concentrated way than citrate, we prefer to use the former for emergencies or hospitalized patients in order to achieve an optimal efficacy. Due to its half life of 4–6 h, its use for outpatients is limited. For these patients citrate appears to be the choice for anticoagulant, though ACD, which is generally used in a 1:8 ratio, also contributes

Table I. Comparison of blood cell separators during plasma exchange therapy

	Discontinuous		Continuous flow centrifugation			
	flow system	N	Earlier model	N	New generation	N
Plasma volume	2.5*	148	4.2	4	2.0	82
Exchanged (L)	(0.8–6.7)**		(3.5–5.0)		(1–5)	
Blood flow (ml/min)						
veno-venous	61	138	60	4	52	78
	(20–100)		(25–90)		(30–100)	
arterio-venous	146	10	–	–	160	4
	(120–180)		–	–	(100–200)	
Plasma flow (ml/min)						
veno-venous	–	–	36.3	4	30	78
	–	–	(10–70)		(10–60)	
arterio-venous	–	–	–	–	90	4
	–	–	–	–	(50–145)	
Length of procedure (min)						
veno-venous	165	138	241	4	87	78
	(65–580)		(175–305)		(44–150)	
arterio-venous	75	10	–	–	30	4
	(65–180)				(20–50)	

* Average ** Range

to the decrease of efficacy due to dilution. This disadvantage may be diminished by increasing both the ratio and the concentration of citrate. Citrate-dependent hypocalcaemia also increases the frequency of moderate side effects and hampers the use of high flow rates. From our experience partial coagulation may occur in the extracorporeal system if citrate is used exclusively. The combination of both low-dosage heparin (generally 2500 IU given i. v. prior to the run) and citrate anticoagulant appears to be an easy way to eliminate this rare problem.

An optimal quality of the cell plasma separation is prerequisite for an optimal quality of the plasma-exchange therapy. As could be anticipated, we did not find any significant retention of plasma proteins [2], including those of high molecular weight, when the separated plasma and that of the input line were compared. Heparin was used for anticoagulation without essential dilution. Since we could not find a decrease of efficacy even after a prolonged period i. e. up to five hours, centrifugal systems appear to be well suited for the application of succeeding techniques, like selective or specific absorption, thereby replacing the plasma-exchange therapy.

The function of cellular blood components has not been reported to be impaired following plasma exchange with centrifugal procedures. A decrease of platelets passing through the machine, now decreased to about 10% as compared to earlier reports, appears to be due to dilution rather than centrifugation.

There is general agreement that side effects of technical origin are rare when centrifugal systems are used. This correlates with our own experience showing that among 354 plasma exchanges performed, only 3 side effects were of potential technical origin (table II). They occurred during the introduction of the discontinuous machines, when the appropriate experience with the volume balance in these systems, known to require special attention, was still lacking. All other side effects were attributable to either the exchange fluid, anticoagulant, immunosuppression, or the underlying disease. From our experience the rate of side effects also depends on the volume of each plasma exchange. We observed nearly twice the number of problems if a volume was exchanged which exceeded twice the plasma volume of the patient. Since alternatively the efficacy of the single exchange decreases with increasing exchange volume [4], we decided upon using frequent, small-volume exchanges rather than rare high-volume therapies. This concept also includes kinetic considerations for the pathogenic material: as an equilibrium in the distribution of protein-bound substances between the circulatory and the extracirculatory compartments can be anticipated, an increase of such material in the patient's plasma can be expected within 24 h or earlier. If the substance to be removed is a protein, for instance an antibody, the production rate also has to be taken into consideration; less for the single exchange, but mainly for a series of therapies. Depending on the specific character of the treated

Table II. Side effects of 354 plasma exchange therapies: Assessment of origin

Origin	Frequency	%
Technical	3	0.8
Exchange fluid	27	7.6
(anaphylaxis, shaking chills. fever, pruritus)		
Anticoagulation	10	2.8
(hypocalcemia)		
Immunosuppression	1	0.3
(infection)		
Underlying disease	4	1.1
(insufficient medication, rise of blood pressure)		

disease, the protein production may be self-limiting, thus terminating during a course of therapies, or may be unaltered or increased, leading to a rebound phenomenon, if no additional medication which depresses the production rate is applied. The production rate thus determines the sequence and frequency of the exchanges. With these considerations in mind we designed a scheme which, if a patient is not vitally endangered, employs 3 plasma exchange therapies of approximately 1–1.5 the patient's plasma volume on 3 consecutive days, 6 therapies with a slightly decreased volume every second day, 6 treatments twice a week and further therapies depending on the specific need, defined by either clinical or laboratory parameters.

Naturally this concept is only a working basis which needs to be adjusted according to the patient's disease and the individual situation. On the other hand, this concept decreased the side effects from over 50% down to 2,5% in the middle of 1980. Since then we had to learn that difficulties resulting from the underlying disease were also of some importance. This increased the rate of side effects to 12,6%.

Filtration has been claimed to be a technical alternative to the plasma separation using centrifugal methods. From our experimental experience with hollow fiber systems so far available for clinical use and having established optimal centrifugal methods, we could not decide whether or not we should introduce filters into the daily clinical routine. We found the following arguments supporting our decision not to use filters:
(1) Due to the formation of secondary membranes a decrease of efficacy is observed with time.
(2) High molecular weight proteins, as for instance circulating immune complexes, are partially retained; the higher the molecular weight, the more.
(3) Since the results of plasma separation are considerably better at high-flow rates of 100 ml–200 ml, there is a tendency to use an unusual access to the circulation with an increased, but unnecessary risk for the patient.
(4) Hemolysis may frequently occur at an increased transmembrane pressure.
(5) The costs of the modules are unusually high (tentimes that of centrifugal systems).

Again, this refers to the standard of those modules so far available for clinical use. Alternatively the experimental development in this field is so fast that improvements, which will lead to a full competition with the centrifugal systems, may be anticipated. We hope to learn at this meeting that flat-sheet membrane filtration is already competitive and available. Our own *in vitro* experience with improved hollow-fiber modules demonstrates that many of the disadvantages of the modules so far available can be eliminated. We have thus set up standards to be met for the introduction of other technologies (table III).

As plasma exchange is unspecific and unselective and as the efficacy is limited by dilution, further improvement needs to be achieved. It is a major concern that substances, conducive or necessary for the patient, may be lost.

Two ways are being evaluated: the selective but *unspecific* removal of plasma protein-fractions using either absorption or differential filtration; or the *specific* absorption of those substances which are supposed to be eliminated.

The optimal way for a specific elimination of pathogenic protein-bound material appears to be either destruction or specific absorption. Since absorption, using immunological methods, appears to be easy to accomplish, we cooperated with our biochemistry department in the development of a model system [6]. Briefly sheep antibody of low-density lipoprotein was coupled to sepharose and fit into a column. Plasma was then separated by continuous flow centrifugation, using either an Aminco Celltrifuge of an IBM Model 2997, and passed through the column. The patient's low-density lipoprotein was thus removed from the plasma. So far this treatment was without any side effects for the patients, but lead to a significant decrease of LDL (fig. 1), which will be described in detail in the following presentation.

From the latest developments reported in the literature and from our

Table III. Cell-plasma separation requirements for optimal plasma exchange therapy

Efficacy	1. No retention of total plasma protein
	2. No retention of plasma components (high molecular weight proteins)
	3. No decrease of efficacy during the separation therapy at any flow rate
Flow rate	30–100 (–300) ml/min
Access to the	*Normal:* Veno-venous or venous (single needle)
circulation	*Only exceptionally:* Arterio-venous or central-venous
Anticoagulants	Several alternatives (heparin, citrate, heparin-citrate)
Safety	No cell damage
	Minimal cell loss
	Extracorporal volume less than 400 ml
Costs	Disposables less than US $ 40.–

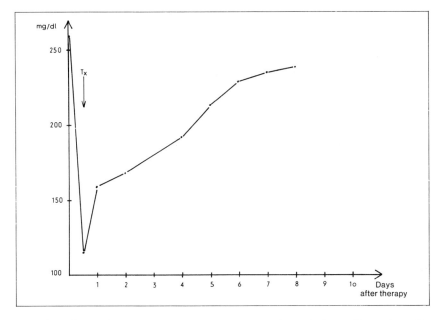

Fig. 1. Specific immunoabsorption ex vivo: Kinetics of total cholesterol in a patient with hypercholesterinemia as a parameter for the LDL-kinetics.

own experience, we conclude that plasma-exchange therapy will be replaced by selective or specific filtration or absorption techniques. At the present time, it is difficult to predict which of the succeeding methods is best for certain diseases, but it appears to be, at least for some diseases, more an economical than a technical problem.

References

1   Abel, J. J.; Rowntree, L. G.; Turner, B. B.: Plasma removal with return of corpuscles (Plasmapheresis). J. Pharmac. exp. Ther. *5:* 625 (1913–14).
2   Borberg, H.: Comparison of cell-plasma separation with different centrifuge techniques. ASAHI-symposium on plasma exchange (Cologne, June 1980).
3   Buckner, C. D.; Clift, R.; Thomas, E. D.: Plasma exchange with the NCI-IBM blood cell separator. Rev. fr. Etud. clin. biol. *14:* 803 (1969).
4   Collins, J. A.: Problems associated with the massive transfusion of stored blood. Surgery *75:* 274 (1974).
5   Graw, R. G.; Buckner, C. D.; Eisel, R.: Plasma exchange transfusion for hepatic coma. New technique. Transfusion *10:* 26 (1970).

6   Stoffel, W.; Demant, T.; Sieberth, H. G.; Borberg, H.; Glöckner, W. M.: Selective removal of Apo-B containing serum lipoproteins from blood plasma. ASAHI-Symposium on plasma exchange (Cologne, June 1980).

Dr. H. Borberg, Medizin. Univ.-Klinik Köln, Labor für Tumorimmunologie, Joseph-Stelzmann-Str. 9, D-5000 Köln 41

Continuous Extracorporeal Immunoadsorption

A Tool for the Selective Removal of Plasma Components.
Low Density Lipoprotein (LDL) Depletion of a
Hypercholesterolemic Patient

W. Stoffel[1], V. Greve[1], J. Lange[1], H. Borberg[2]

[1] Institut für Physiologische Chemie Köln, FRG
[2] Medizinische Klinik der Universität Köln, FRG

A concept and its experimental realization in a collaborative study are presented which permit the highly selective removal of any blood plasma component from endogenous or exogenous sources, provided they have antigenic or haptenic properties.

Our primary goal was the selective removal of low density serum lipoprotein which would lead to the reduction of plasma cholesterol, an event most desirable in homo- and heterozygous familial hypercholesterolemia.

So far, surgical intervention, such as ileal bypass [1] and terminal portacaval shunt [2–4], and nonsurgical procedures such as plasmapheresis [5, 6] or the discontinuous venous blood removal, adsorption of VLDL and LDL to heparin sepharose and reinfusion of the filtered blood [7] are being used. In the latter experiments, plasma-cholesterol levels were lowered by 15–20% in the rather expensive plasma-exchange experiments of *Thompson et al.* [5] and in *Apstein et al.* [6] a decrease of 60% was achieved. The present cost of a plasma exchange in the U. S. amounts to $ 800. The disadvantage due to these economic considerations and the necessity of continued treatment for an indefinite period are apparent.

The concept is as follows:

(1) The procedure for the removal of a plasma component must be highly specific.

(2) The method must be capable of continuously depleting the plasma of the component under study.

(3) The method must be rapid and efficient, e. g. eventually leading to a complete removal of the component.

(4) The physical status of the individual should remain unimpaired.

(5) A repetitive use should make the system financially feasible.

The example reported here, namely the LDL removal from swine plasma, should prove the potential of the procedure, the methodology of which will be reported in details elsewhere [8].

The highly specific removal is achieved by immunoadsorption: Serum-LDL was purified exhaustively for

(a) the covalent coupling to sepharose CL-4B, and

(b) for the immunization of sheep.

Sheep anti-LDL was adsorbed by the LDL-Sepharose and desorbed with glycine buffer, pH 2.8, as monospecific antibodies after thorough elution of the non-immunoadsorbed plasma proteins with PBS (phosphatebuffered saline). 3–4 g of monospecific anti-LDL-IgG were isolated and covalently cross-linked to CNBr-activated Sepharose CL-4B. This anti-LDL-Sepharose-4B bed was used as a selective adsorber of LDL from the plasma.

Pigs develop a form of arteriosclerosis somewhat resembling that of humans [9].

It can be induced experimentally by a number of methods [10]. Therefore a swine is the most rewarding experimental animal, particularly under the conditions reported in this cooperative study.

We proceeded as follows:

Silicon tubings of 2 mm internal diameter were introduced into the common carotoid artery, the jugular vein, or the femoral artery and vein of the 25 to 40 kg deeply anesthetized pigs.

Into the arteriovenous or venous-venous shunt a continous-flow blood centrifuge (model Aminco celltrifuge) was interposed to separate the plasma from any corpuscular elements and the erythrocytes, white

---

Fig. 1. Schematic diagram of the arrangement of continuous-flow centrifuge (Aminco ▷ celltrifuge) and immunoadsorbent column in the shunt.

Fig. 2. Kinetics of LDL removal from normal pig plasma in vivo by adsorption to anti-LDL-Sepharose CL-4B.

Curve (a): Protein concentration as marker for dilutional effects

Curve (b): LDL concentration during an immunoadsorption experiment

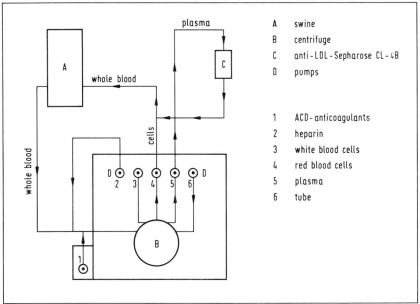

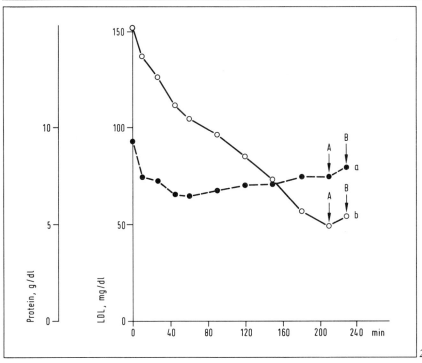

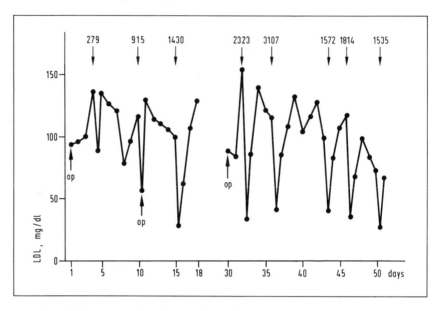

Fig. 3. LDL concentration of a normal pig after repeated immunoadsorption treatment. Op: operation of arterio – venous or venous – venous shunt. Numbers above arrows: LDL (mg) desorbed from immunoadsorption column after experiment.

cells, and thrombocyte concentrate. The plasma was passed over a Sepharose 4B-LDL-antibody column (fig. 1). Its capacity is sufficient to adsorb about 5 g total LDL-cholesterol corresponding to 11 g of low-density lipoproteins.

The LDL-depleted plasma eluting from the LDL-adsorber is recombined with the erythrocyte-concentrate flow before entering the venous side of the shunt.

In more than 35 experiments with normal pigs we were able to demonstrate

(1) that our approach selectively removes the apo-B-containing lipoproteins LDL and VLDL;

(2) that the repeated application of this highly selective immunoadsorption method is tolerated without any physical impairment.

The following figures analyse the biochemical parameters:

Figure 2 depicts the kinetics of the removal of LDL during the experiments.

Figure 3 outlines some features characteristic for the experimental animal:

(a) The transient influence of the shunt operation on plasma LDL-concentration of the animal which normalizes within 2–4 days.
(b) In some experiments an 'overshoot' phenomenon was observed, following the establishment of the pre-experimental LDL levels after immunoadsorption, which occurs within 4–8 days [3–6].
(c) Repetitive experiments show identical kinetics.
(d) Serum enzymes, electrolytes, urea, creatine, glucose, and several hematological parameters remain unaltered with the exception of the lowered hematocrit, due to the removal of several blood samples for analysis during the experiment.

Hypercholesterolemic swines with total serum LDL-cholesterol of 600 mg/dl due to a 2% cholesterol diet over a period of almost one year were used. For this LDL-adsorption two anti-LDL-columns were arranged in series and used alternately. The column completely saturated with LDL was regenerated with glycine, HCl, pH 2.8 buffer, and neu-

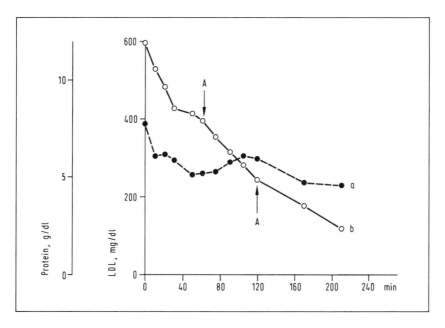

Fig. 4. Kinetics of LDL removal from hypercholesterolemic swine in vivo by adsorption to anti-LDL-Sepharose CL-4B.
A: Change to regenerated anti-LDL-column
Curve (a): Protein concentration
Curve (b): LDL concentration during experiment

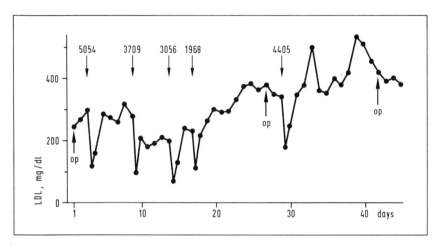

Fig. 5. LDL concentration of a hypercholesterolemic pig after repeated treatment to immunoadsorption.
Op: Shunt operation. Numbers above arrows: LDL (mg) desorbed from immunoadsorption column.

tralized with PBS, while the second column was in function. As demonstrated in figure 4, LDL levels were lowered from 600 to 120 mg/dl. The kinetics of the replacement of the LDL-concentration was comparable to that of a normal swine (fig. 5).

Approved by the ethic commission of our university's medical faculty we then started an immunoadsorption treatment of a 29-year-old hypercholesterolemic volunteer.

A venous-venous shunt between the cubital veins of the patient was used for the extracorporeal blood centrifugation and the immunoad-

Table I. Results of three LDL-immunoadsorption treatments of a 29-year-old hypercholesterolemic male volunteer

Experiment	LDL/VLDL cholesterol concentration before experiment (mg/dl)	LDL/VLDL cholesterol concentration after experiment (mg/dl)	LDL/VLDL cholesterol removed (%)	LDL/VLDL cholesterol removed (mg)	Plasma-volume passed on column (l)
I	220	80	63,6	4654	5,4
II	254	102	59,8	3782	4,0
III	182	77	57,7	3032	4,2

sorber. Table I summarizes the results of three treatments all of which occurred without the slightest physical impairment to the patient.

Figure 6 outlines the kinetics of the patient's LDL-concentration in these successive experiments.

Figure 7 summarizes the results of this new approach for the removal of a plasma component; in this case the apo-B-containing lipoproteins are positively correlated to the pathogenesis of arteriosclerosis.

(1) LDL can be specifically removed during a short-time (2–4 h) application by our set-up.

(2) The LDL-concentration returns to the original level within 2–3 weeks. The method is, therefore, acceptable for repeated and routine application, particularly in homozygotes.

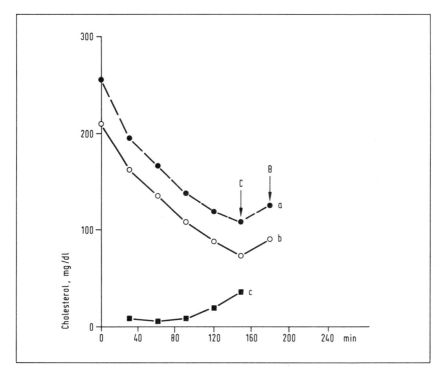

Fig. 6. Kinetics of LDL removal from a hypercholesterolemic male volunteer by adsorption to anti-LDL-Sepharose CL-4B.
Curve (a): Total cholesterol concentration
Curve (b): LDL/VLDL cholesterol concentration
Curve (c): LDL/VLDL cholesterol concentration (sample after column).

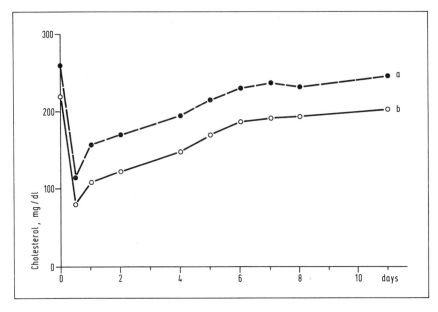

Fig. 7. LDL depletion in extracorporeal combined plasma separation, immunoadsorption and kinetic of LDL replenishment of plasma LDL in man.
Curve (a): Total cholesterol
Curve (b): LDL/VLDL cholesterol

(3) No 'overshoot-synthesis' was observed in man.

The potential of the method is obvious

(a) for biochemical questions such as: Is the gradual increase of LDL after its removal to the original level due to a de novo synthesis of the lipid and apoprotein components of LDL or are cholesterol deposits mobilized by the dramatic changes of serum-cholesterol concentrations?

(b) since the principle of this approach appears to be adaptable to other clinical problems, basically to the selective removal of plasma components with antigenic sites.

Finally returning to the conceptual basis of our approach outlined in the beginning. We are confident that this method may be of great benefit to removing the main-risk factor of coronary heart disease of homo- and heterozygous hypercholesterolemic patients.

The treatment of a female homozygous familial hypercholesteremic patient is in progress.

References

1 Thompson, G. R.; Gotto, A. M.: Ileal bypass in the treatment of hyperlipoproteinaemia. Lancet *i:* 35–36 (1973).
2 Starzl, T. E.; Chase, H. P.; Putnam, C. W.; Porter, K. A.: Portacaval shunt in hyperlipoproteinaemia. Lancet *i:* 940–944 (1973).
3 Starzl, T. E.; Chase, H. P.; Putnam, C. W.; Nore, J. J.; Farnell, R. H. Jr.; Porter, K. A.: Portacaval shunt in hyperlipoproteinaemia. Lancet *ii:* 1263 (1974).
4 Stein, T. E.; Mieny, C.; Spitz, L.: Portacaval shunt in four patients with homozygous hypercholesterolaemia. Lancet *i:* 832–835 (1975).
5 Thompson, G. R.; Lowenthal, R.; Myant, N. B.: Plasma exchange in the management of homozygous familial hypercholesterolaemia. Lancet *i:* 1208–1211 (1975).
6 Apstein, C. S.; Zilversmit, D. B.; George, P. K.; Lees, R. S.: Effect of intensive plasmapheresis on the plasma-cholesterol concentration with familial hypercholesterolemia. Arteriosclerosis *31:* 105–115 (1978).
7 Lupien, P. J.; Moorjani, S.; Awad, J.: A new approach to the management of familial hypercholesterolaemia: Removal of plasma cholesterol based on the principle of affinity chromatography. Lancet *ii:* 1261–1265 (1976).
8 Stoffel, W.; Demant, Th.: Selective removal of apolipoprotein B-containing serum-lipoproteins from blood plasma. Proc. natn. Acad. Sci. USA *78:* 611–615 (1981).
9 Rowsell, H. C.; Mustard, J. F.; Downie, H. G.: Experimental atherosclerosis in swine. Ann. N. Y. Acad. Sci. *127:* 743–762 (1965).
10 Marshall, M.: Atherogenese: Experimentelle Untersuchungen zur Pathogenese obliterierender Arteriopathien am Miniaturschwein. Münch. med. Wschr. *121:* 1211–1218 (1979).

Volker Greve, Institut für Physiologische Chemie der Universität Köln, Joseph-Stelzmann-Str. 52, D–5000 Köln 41

A Comparative Study
of the Efficacy of Two Methods of Plasmapheresis:
Centrifugation with ACD or Heparin
and Membrane Filtration with Two Different
Cellulose Diacetate Hollow-Fiber Membranes

P. Rawer, K.-H. Sommerlad, K. Goretzky, H. W. Leber

Zentrum für Innere Medizin der Justus Liebig-Universität, Giessen, FRG

Introduction

In view of the latest developments in plasma exchange treatment, the following general questions arise:

(1) In which illnesses is treatment by plasma exchange indicated?
(2) Does the efficacy of plasmapheresis differ depending on the method used (centrifugation – membrane filtration)?
(3) How much plasma should be exchanged, how often, and for how long?
(4) Is it possible to selectively eliminate substances which cause or sustain an illness?

The application of plasmapheresis has been increasing over the last 3 years in therapy for various nephrologic and neurologic illnesses, in which immunomechanisms are suspected to play a role or else have been verified etiologically, as well as in endocrinologically triggered metabolic illnesses and intoxications [1]. On the basis of previous investigations [2, 3], Goodpasture's syndrome and myasthenia gravis are clearly indications for plasmapheresis; however, the indication for all other illnesses must be supported by controlled studies. Currently, the decision of how much, how often, and how long plasma should be exchanged depends on the therapist's intuition, since in most instances the substance to be eliminated is unknown, and kinetic investigations are not yet available. Consequently, even a selective elimination is only feasible when the illness to be treated by plasmapheresis can be attributed to the presence of one or more toxic substances.

The following investigations deal with the difference in efficacy of plasmapheresis by centrifugation and by membrane filtration. This difference was derived from the elimination rate of immunoglobulins, inflammation mediators, and other plasma proteins with different molecular weights. Furthermore, we report on the possibility of selectively removing antibodies to DNA and motor end-plates from the separated plasma of patients who underwent plasma exchange. Also the elimination of immune complexes produced in vitro and containing immunoglobulin-G by means of immobilized protein A is discussed.

Methods

Plasma separation by means of centrifugation was carried out with the Haemonetics, model 30, which was equipped with a 225 ml rotor. For separation by membrane filtration we used two plasma capillary filters (Plasmaflo 01 and Plasmaflo 02, the successor product of Asahi, Japan) on a hemoprocessor (Sartorius, FRG). In both procedures the plasma exchange volume amounted to 3 l; the substitution solution was 3% human albumin/electrolyte/glucose solution. In the centrifugation method, anticoagulation was achieved with either ACD or heparin; for membrane filtration only heparin was used. With the centrifugation method, blood-flow rates between 70 and 120 ml/min were obtained; in membrane filtration the blood flow remained constant at 200 ml/min. The transmembrane pressure in the case of the latter method was between 50 and 100 mmHg. Plasma exchange treatment with centrifugation or membrane filtration was applied to various illnesses (rapidly progressive glomerulonephritis, myasthenia gravis, membranoproliferative glomerulonephritis, amyotrophic lateral sclerosis, hyperlipoproteinemia with terminal renal insufficiency, Goodpasture's syndrome, panarteriitis nodosa, membranous glomerulopathy, Wegener's granulomatosis, and plasmacytoma). According to the principle of radial immunodiffusion (Partigen, Behringwerke, Marburg/FRG), we quantified the different plasma proteins, such as α_1-antitrypsin, transferrin, C3, C4, IgG, IgA, IgM, fibrinogen, α_2-macroglobulin, β-lipoprotein. The colloid osmotic pressure was determined with the Weil-Onkometersystem 186 (Instr. Lab. Int.,

Lexington/USA). Sepharose and protein-A Sepharose-CL4B was obtained from the Pharmacia Company (Uppsala/Sweden) and used in the batch and perfusion system. Antinuclear factors, anti-DNA (both single- and double-stranded) were assayed by Dr. Helmke (Med. Poliklinik, Justus Liebig-Universität, Giessen/FRG) by immunofluorescence and radioimmunoassay. The immune complexes were determined by laser nephelometry together with Dr. Hobler (Med. Poliklinik, Justus Liebig-Universität, Giessen/FRG). Dr. J. Sondac (Zentrallaboratorium des Blutspendedienstes der Niederlande, Red Cross, Amsterdam) determined the antibodies to motor end-plates by an immunofluorescence technique using α-BuTx. To compare the efficacy of the two plasma separation procedures, the elimination coefficient was calculated (quotient of concentration of a substance in pooled plasma or filtrate and the baseline concentration). For statistical evaluation the χ-test as modified by *Van der Waerden* [4] was used.

Results

The elimination coefficients for various plasma proteins with molecular weights between 50,000 and 950,000 are shown in figure 1 for both the centrifugation method with ACD as anticoagulant and for the membrane filtration method with Plasmaflo 01. The centrifugation method is significantly superior as regards the elimination of α_1-antitrypsin, transferrin, IgG, IgA, C3, C4, fibrinogen, and IgM. There is no significant difference between the two methods for α_2-macroglobulin. The mean elimination coefficient for centrifugation is 0.57; for membrane filtration it is 0.32.

Two cellulose diacetate hollow-fiber filters were investigated: the Plasmaflo 01 with an internal capillary diameter of 370 μm, an external diameter of 700 μm, and an effective surface area of 0.65 m²; and a second filter (Plasmaflo 02) differs essentially from 01 through its reduced membrane thickness (75 μm) and reduced effective surface area (0.5 m²).

Figure 2 shows the elimination coefficients derived with the filters Plasmaflo 01 and 02 for the above-mentioned plasma proteins. The majority of the investigated proteins (α1-antitrypsin, transferrin, IgG, IgA, fibrinogen, and IgM) are eliminated significantly better when Plasmaflo 02 is used. The mean elimination coefficient for Plasmaflo 02 is 0.52 as opposed to 0.32 for Plasmaflo 01.

If plasma separation with centrifugation is carried out on the

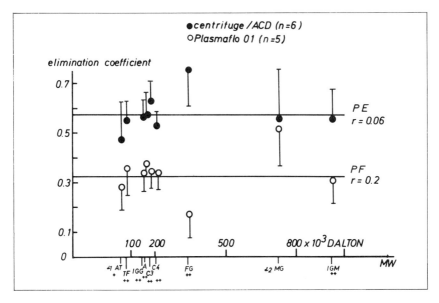

Fig. 1. Comparison of efficacy with the centrifugation method/ACD and membrane filtration (Plasmaflo 01). α_1-Antitrypsin (α1-AT), transferrin (TF), complement factor C3 (C3), complement factor C4 (C4), fibrinogen (FG), IgG, IgA (A), IgM, α_2-macroglobulin (α_2-MG). Probability of error $=0.5\%:++$; $=1\%:+$.

Haemonetics machine, the eliminated plasma is diluted due to the continual addition of ACD (the pump ratio between the blood pump and the anticoagulant pump remains constant). With a hematocrit of 42%, 3,000 ml of eliminated plasma contains approximately 750ml ACD. To cancel this dilution effect, we carried out centrifugation with heparin (30,000 units/separation) without addition of ACD. A comparison of the elimination coefficients of the above-cited plasma proteins is shown in figure 3 for membrane filtration (Plasmaflo 02) and centrifugation with heparin. Centrifugation yields a higher elimination coefficient for all plasma proteins examined; its mean value is 0.64 compared with 0.52 for membrane filtration. However, the differences were significant only for the complement factor C3 and for IgM. Figure 3 further shows that β-lipoproteins with a molecular weight of about 2,400,000 have an elimination coefficient that corresponds to that of plasma proteins. Here is no significant difference between the two methods.

Protein-A, a staphylococcic protein with the property of binding selectively to immunoglobulin-G [5, 6], is suitable for selective elimina-

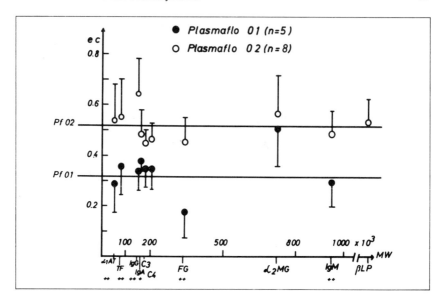

Fig. 2. Comparison of efficacy with two capillary filters (Plasmaflo 01 and Plasmaflo 02) on the basis of elimination coefficients for different plasma proteins (see fig. 1).

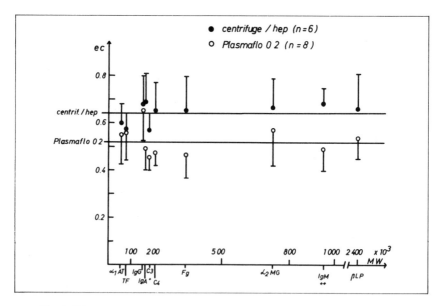

Fig. 3. Elimination coefficients for different plasma proteins with centrifugation and heparin or membrane filtration with Plasmaflo 02.

tion from separated plasma. An immobilized protein-A on Sepharose-CL4B was studied in batch and single-pass procedures for its binding capacity to pathologic immunoglobulins. In the batch experiment, the separated plasma of a patient with lupus erythematosus was incubated with 3ml protein-A Sepharose-CL4B or control Sepharose. Compared with control Sepharose, a reduction of the DNA-antibody titer ratio from 1:80 to 0 is possible with protein-A Sepharose. Also the antinuclear factors can be reduced from a baseline titer ratio of 1:80 to 1:10. Likewise antibodies to native DNA were reduced from 73% to 20% (fig. 4).

After 25ml plasma of a patient with myasthenia gravis with identifiable antibodies to motor end-plates had passed through a column filled with 5ml protein-A Sepharose-CL4B, a reduction of the baseline titer (0:80) was achieved by 1–2 titer steps in comparison with the control Sepharose (determination was made in 5ml outflowing fractions, fig. 5).

As shown in previous investigations [7], immune complexes formed in vitro from human albumin and albumin-antibody serum from rabbits can likewise be removed by immobilized protein-A.

Discussion

On the basis of the calculated elimination coefficients for different plasma proteins with molecular weights between 50,000 and 950,000, the unequivocal superiority of centrifugation over the membrane filtration method carried out with Plasmaflo 01 was demonstrated, especially with regard to the elimination capacity for the immunoglobulins IgG, IgA, IgM, and inflammation mediators such as fibrinogen, complement factors C3 and C4. Compared to Plasmaflo 01 we found better elimination rates with the successor product Plasmaflo 02. These rates were significantly higher for the immunoglobulins IgG, IgA, and IgM. A comparison of this new membrane with the traditional method of centrifugation with ACD as anticoagulant showed no significant differences as regards elimination efficacy for the immunoglobulins IgG, IgA, and IgM. If plasma separation by centrifugation is carried out with heparin and without ACD, higher elimination coefficients for the examined plasma proteins are obtained since the dilution effect is absent. A comparison of plasma separation with membrane filtration using Plasmaflo 02 and centrifugation using heparin showed a significant difference in favor of centrifugation only for the complement factor C3 and for IgM. However, the immunoglobulins IgG

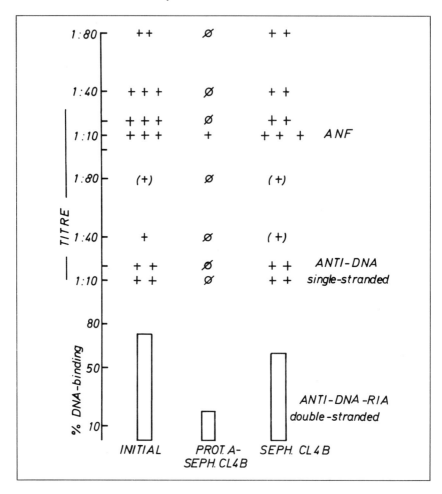

Fig. 4. Batch test for selective elimination of antinuclear factors, antibodies to denaturized DNA (single stranded) and native DNA (double strand) by means of protein-A Sepharose-CL4B. Values were determined before and after incubation of 5 ml of patient's plasma for 20 min with 3 ml moist Sepharose.

and A, complement factor C4, fibrinogen, and also α_1-antitrypsin, transferrin, and α_2-macroglobulin are eliminated to the same extent by both methods. This is also true for the elimination of β-lipoproteins, a molecule with molecular weight of 2,400,000 due to its lipid content. Thus, the efficacy of the new filter capillaries is considerably better than that of the membrane filters previously available, and they are comparable to that of

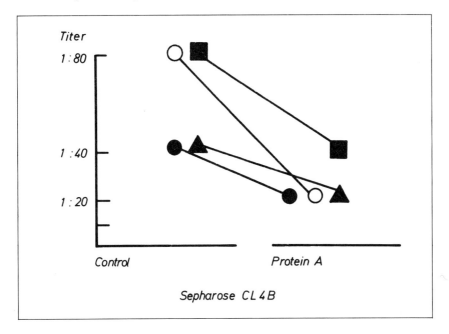

Fig. 5. In vitro column perfusion of 5 ml protein-A Sepharose with 5 x 5 ml plasma from a patient with myasthenia gravis with antibodies to motor end-plates: flow rate = 1 ml/min.

the centrifugation method, at least for the majority of the proteins investigated.

Both plasma separation methods involve nonspecific elimination principles with the unavoidable loss of physiologic plasma components (e. g., coagulation factors, albumin). Thus, these factors must be substituted (at least albumin), a process that is costly as well as risky (transmission of hepatitis). Consequently, a selective elimination of the pathologic factors would be desirable. Such a procedure should endeavor to return the physiologic blood components to the patient after primary plasma separation. The selective elimination of antibodies or immune complexes is recommended for diseases proved to be caused by pathologic immunoglobulins or immune complexes, e.g., myasthenia gravis with antibodies to motor end-plates or Goodpasture's syndrome with antiglomerular basement membrane antibodies, and glomerulonephritis with circulating immune complexes. That a selective elimination of pathologic antibodies is possible was shown by the in vitro experiments with immobilized protein-A.

Summary

In principle, plasma-exchange therapy can be carried out by means of centrifugation or membrane filtration. The former was performed using ACD or heparin; membrane filtration was applied with two different cellulose diacetate hollow-fiber filters. To compare their elimination efficacy, we determined the elimination coefficient of various plasma proteins (α_1-antitrypsin, transferrin, IgG, IgA, IgM, C3, C4, fibrinogen, α_2-macroglobulin, and β-lipoprotein). Whereas membrane filtration with the filter Plasmaflo 01 is clearly inferior as regards elimination capacity to that of centrifugation, the successor product (Plasmaflo 02) shows considerably improved efficacy and is comparable to the centrifugation method. In vitro experiments with immobilized protein-A show that, in principle, the selective elimination of pathologic antibodies, e.g., antibodies to motor end-plates or DNA antibodies from separated plasma, is possible.

References

1 Lockwood, C. M.: An overview. Plasma Ther. *1:* 1–12 (1979).
2 Lockwood, C. M.; Peters, D. K.: The role of plasma exchange and immunosuppression in the treatment of Goodpasture's syndrome and glomerulonephritis. Plasma Ther. *1:* 19–27 (1979).
3 Newsom-Davis, J.: Plasma exchange in myasthenia gravis. Plasma Ther. *2:* 17–32 (1979).
4 Van der Waerden, B. L.; Nievergelt, E.: Tafeln zum Vergleich zweier Stichproben mittels χ-Test und Zeichentest (Springer-Verlag, Berlin 1956).
5 Kronvall, G.; Williams, R. C.: Differences in anti-protein-A activity among IgG-subgroups. J. Immun. *103:* 828–833 (1969).
6 Morgan, M. R. A.; Johnson, P. M.; Dihn, P. D. G.: Electrophoretic desorption of immunoglobulins from immobilized protein-A and other ligands. J. immunol. Methods *23:* 381 (1978).
7 Rawer, P.; Sommerlad, K.; Goretzki, K.; Leber, H. W.: Elimination of plasma proteins during plasma separation using either centrifugation or membrane filtration and selective removal of immunoglobulin-G and immune-complexes with immobilized protein-A. In: Sieberth (ed.), Plasma Exchange, pp. 65–70 (Schattauer-Verlag, Stuttgart 1980).

Dr. P. Rawer, Zentrum für Innere Medizin, Klinikstr. 36, D–6300 Giessen

Targeted Elimination of Plasma Proteins: Cascade Filtration (Immunoadsorption and Affinity Adsorption)

H. G. Sieberth, W. M. Glöckner, H. Kierdorf, W. Stoffel, C. Dienst

Med. Univ.-Klinik Köln, FRG

By using membranes or the cell centrifuge it is possible to separate large quantities of plasma from blood-cells in a short time. In plasma-exchange treatment in its present form, the separated plasma is usually discarded in toto and is replaced by albumin solutions or foreign plasma. Many attempts are being made towards removing solely the pathogenic substances from the separated plasma so that the remainder of the plasma can be reinfused to the patient. In many illnesses, for which plasma exchange has been described as an effective treatment, we do not yet even know whether the process removes any toxic substances, and certainly not which toxic substances these might be.

If we were to succeed in isolating defined groups of substances from the plasma, we would certainly also be able to gain new information about these – still hypothetical – substances.

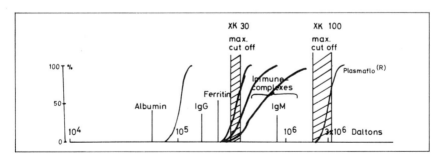

Fig. 1. Spectrum of individual proteins and possible separation bands for cascade filtration.

Although direct removal of these substances from the blood would certainly be the most elegant method, the indirect route via plasma will, in many cases, still be the method initially chosen to avoid possible damage to the blood cells. Of the processes currently available, cascade filtration, immunoadsorption, and affinity adsorption are the most important for targeted elimination of plasma proteins. I would like to limit my discussion here mainly to those methods which have already been used in practice on humans or on experimental animals.

Cascade Filtration

If the plasma is passed through several filters with differing pore sizes, the separated plasma can be split into fractions of differing molecular-weight ranges. The fraction which is expected to contain the highest proportion of pathogenic substances is then discarded and the remanining plasma fractions are retransfused. In the first stage of cascade filtration, called membrane-plasma separation, the blood cells are separated from the plasma. This stage corresponds to cell separation using a cell centrifuge.

In the second stage, called plasma filtration, high-molecular proteins are separated from low-molecular proteins (fig. 1). The filtrate from this stage can either be fed straight back into the bloodstream or can be further processed in a third stage. The recirculation of the non-separated plasma through the second stage causes the protein concentration in the circulating plasma to increase and the protein concentration in the filtrate to decrease. To prevent the protein concentration from increasing the circulating plasma must be diluted to a sufficient extent. This, however, means that the diluted plasma from stage 2 must be subsequently reduced in stage 3 in volume by removing water and electrolytes (fig. 2).

The difficulty at present lies in obtaining filters with an adequate flow throughput and a defined cut-off point. The membrane-plasma separators commercially available at present have a cut-off point at approx. 3×10^6 Dalton. Membranes of similar structure (i.e. structured like a network) and a lower cut-off point are currently being tested for use in cascade filtration. Such filters have already succeeded in separating IgM, whose molecular weight is in the same range as those of the circulating immune complexes [13]. It has not yet proved possible to cleanly separate albumin and IgG by using membrane modules. The problem here is probably due

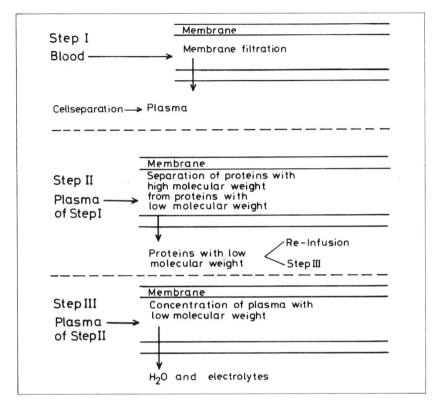

Fig. 2. Cascade filtration with several cascades.

to the fact that the statistical spread of pore size in these membranes is too great. Nuclear track-etched membranes with a well-defined pore diameter [9] and only a small statistical spread have already been used for membrane filtration of blood [11], but are not yet available for cascade filtration.

In vivo cascade filtration using two membranes has been carried out on humans [1] and on dogs [13]. By means of double-filtration plasmapheresis with polyvinylalcohol and ethylenevinyl hollow-fiber membranes, *Agishi et al.* were able to increase the albumin/globulin ratio from 1.8 to 2.5 in the reinfused plasma.

Malchesky et al. [8] have removed cryoglobulins from plasma by double filtration as *Dr. Gurland* has already mentioned. The plasma obtained from membrane-plasma separation was cooled in an ice-bath, which caused the cryoglobulins to precipitate. The gelled cryoglobulins were separated from the rest of the plasma by using the same membrane in a second step.

After testing the cascade-filtration process in vitro and animal experiments, we have now started using it on humans. Two cellulose diacetate

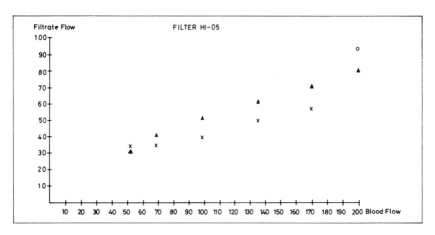

Fig. 3. Relationship between blood-flow rate and quantity of filtrate for the Hi-05 membrane-plasma separator.

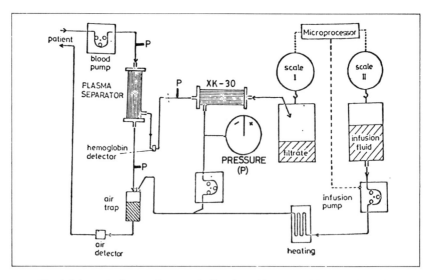

Fig. 4. Schematic diagram for cascade filtration with two modules containing filters of different pore sizes.

modules (Asahi Medical Co., Tokyo) with different cut-off points were used.

The plasma separation was, as usual, carried out with a Haemo-processor® (Sartorius Co., Göttingen). The new filter Hi-05 was used to separate the plasma. This filter allows large quantities of filtrate to be produced even at low blood-flow rates (fig. 3). Also, the protein concentration in the filtrate is higher than that produced by the Plasmaflo®. The filtrate was fed directly to the filter XK-30-E; the resulting filtrate was then fed back to the bloodstream by means of a pump. The pump-flow rate was adjusted so that the negative pressure never exceeded 50 mm Hg. The plasma which had not been filtered was collected in a microprocessor-controlled balance and was substituted by an equal volume of 3% albumin solution (fig. 4). At a blood-flow rate of approximately 200 ml/min,

Table I. Cascade filtration in humans: Relationship between plasma-flow rate and quantity of filtrate for the XK-30-E filter

T	Blood ml/'	Plasmaseparator Hi 0,5 Filtrate ml/'	Plasmafilter XK 30 E Filtrate ml/'	Final filtrate ml
25'	200	80	40	700
60'	200	89	40	2000
85'	200	80	40	3600

Table II. Cascade filtration in humans: Protein content of the blood, the separated plasma, and the filtered plasma

	Blood 100%	Plasmaseparator Hi 0,5 Filtrate 100%	Plasmafilter XK 30 E Filtrate
Total protein g/dl	3,6	3,0 (84%)	2,7 (93%)
Albumin g/dl	2,2	1,9 (85%)	1,7 (90%)
IgG mg/dl	60	52 (87%)	42 (81%)
IgA mg/dl	58	53 (91%)	40 (75%)
IgM mg/dl	93	38 (41%)	3,5 (9%)

around 80–90 ml/min of plasma was separated. Around 50 % of the separated plasma was filtered once more in the XK-30-E plasma filter. The quantity of filtrate remained almost constant during the 1–1½ h plasma separation (table I). The sieving effect of the filter was markedly lower for IgM than for the other measured proteins. In vitro tests on stored, cooled plasma IgM could not be detected in the filtrate from the XK-30-E [13]. The filters used here in the cascade were still very slightly permeable by IgM (table II).

Immunoadsorption and Affinity Adsorption

It is possible to eliminate selectively a particular pathogenic plasma component if the substance exhibits antigenic or certain types of binding properties. The most highly selective elimination is obtained by immunoadsorption. To do this, the antibodies are bonded by their Fc-fragment onto the surface of fixed or low-mobility phases. In this way *Stoffel et al.* (1980) were able to lower the levels of cholesterol and LDL (low-density lipoproteins) in pigs by using antibodies from sheep directed against pig VLDL (very low-density lipoproteins) and LDL. They have recently succeeded in carrying out similar processes in humans. The purified monospecific antibodies are bonded to CNBr-activated Sepharose CL-4-B. Plasma produced by membrane separation or by the cell centrifuge is fed through immunoadsorption columns filled with anti-LDL Sepharose CL-4-B and then fed back to the blood. This allows the cholesterol and LDL concentrations in the organism to be reduced to 10–20 % of their initial values within 2 h. The bonded LDL can be released from the anti-LDL Sepharose by a glycin-buffer solution of pH 3 and removed from the column. The efficiency of the column remained unchanged after more than 25 cycles of LDL adsorption and desorption. The extracorporeal antigen-antibody reaction was well tolerated by the organism. No clinical indications of an activation of complement system, which was to be feared, could be detected.

Heparin Sepharose CL-4-B was able to achieve a similarly effective removal of LDL.

The bonding of IgG to protein-A is less selective than the antigen-antibody reaction [3]. There is a covalent bonding of the Fc-fragment from human or mammal IgG to protein-A. In this way the IgG in antigen-antibody-complement complexes can also be bonded [6]. Staphylococcus aureus Cowan I, which has protein-A on its surface, is being used by some groups of researchers to extract IgG from the plasma in vivo. Both the removal of the plasma [15] and the isolated elimination of IgG are thought to have an inhibitory effect on tumors. This problem will also be discussed in other papers here. I only wish to mention the technique for isolated removal of IgG. A pure culture of Staphylococcus aureus Cowan I is used. Staphylococci of diameter 10^{-4} cm are prevented from passing into the circulation by membranes with a maximum pore diameter of 2×10^{-5} cm. Various different arrangements of the membranes are used (fig. 5). In the apparatus chosen by *Ray* (1980), the plasma flows by the staphylococci which are outside the membranes. A flow force on the permeable proteins is set up across the membrane. The adsorption of IgG onto the protein-A of the staphylococcus causes a continuous outflow of IgG from the stream of plasma passing through the membrane. The resulting reduction of IgG in the human organism is fairly small, in the order of 10–20 %. In the system chosen by *Terman et al.* (1980), the staphylococci are placed in a chamber which is enclosed by membrane walls and through which the plasma flows. In dogs, a reduction of the IgG-concentration in the circulating plasma of around 40–50 % was achieved. When radioactive tracer-marked staphylococci were used, no parts could be detected as having been carried through the membrane. The majority of the dogs, however, registered a rise in temperature after the treatment.

It is to be expected that a greater amount of IgG could be bound by a more thorough mixing of plasma and staphylococcus. With the Plasmaflo® modules generally used today for membrane-plasma separation, with a pore diameter of 0.2 μm, it should be possible to separate the staphylococci from the plasma.

Purified protein-A can be bonded to Sepharose CL-4-B, and 2 mg of protein-A can adsorb around 25 mg of IgG. In vitro, plasma can be almost completely freed of IgG by using protein-A Sepharose CL-4-B. Assuming that in a plasma-exchange treatment around 40 g of IgG is removed, then calculation shows that this could be bonded by around 3.2 of protein-A. At current prices for protein-A, this 'trapping' process would cost around DM 100,000 (US $ 50,000). By using an acid buffer, IgG can be released from protein-A Sepharose. Sepharose is available in the form of beads with diameters ranging between 200–300 μm, which can be held back by a net with a mesh size of 80 μm. It might be possible, in this way, to remove IgG from the blood directly without plasma separation.

Having given a brief look into the future, I would like to finish by

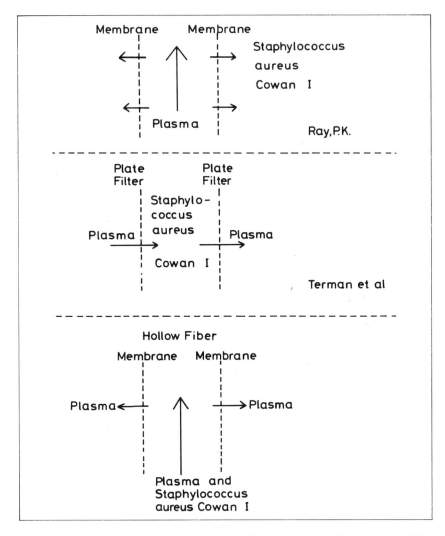

Fig. 5. Arrangement of the membranes and direction of plasma flow for various different methods of eliminating IgA using Staphylococcus aureus Cowan I.

describing two methods which make it possible to eliminate certain substances directly from the blood.

Scharschmidt et al. (1977) perfused albumin-conjugated agarose with the blood of jaundiced rhesus monkeys. One hour of perfusion through four adsorption columns connected in parallel caused a reduction of the bilirubin level to approximately half of its initial value. The major disadvantage of this method is the loss of approximately 60 % of the leukocytes initially present and 90 % of the thrombocytes. Albumin-agarose particles were found histologically in the livers of the animals.

A simple method of removing lipoproteins by bonding them to heparin agarose has been described by *Lupin et al.* (1980). The blood was fed into transfusion bags filled with heparin agarose. At the same time $CaCl_2$ was added. Divalent ions must be present for the lipoproteins to be adsorbed onto the heparin agarose. After some time, the blood was retransfused from the bags. In homozygous familial hypercholesterolemia, this method, which treats 800 ml of blood extracorporeally, succeeded in reducing the plasma cholesterin by about 200 mg/dl. This also markedly reduced the VLDL and the LDL levels, while the level of HDL (high-density lipoproteins), which has a protective effect, remained unchanged. By repeating this treatment at approximately 2-week intervals, the mean cholesterol concentration was in two cases markedly reduced.

Summary

The methods discussed above for the elimination of particular substances from blood or plasma are certainly only of partial relevance to the treatment of malignant growths. These can, however, represent important starting points for the development of new methods.

References:

1   Agishi, T.; Kaneko, J.; Hasuoi, Y.; Sanaka, T.; Ota, K.; Amemika, H.; Sugino, N.: Double filtration plasmapheresis with no or minimal amount of blood derivate for substitution. In: Sieberth (ed.), Plasma Exchange, p. 53 (F. K. Schattauer Verlag, Stuttgart–New York 1980).
2   Bansal, S. C.; Bansal, B. R.; Thoma, H. C.; Siegel, P. D.; Rhodas, J. E.; Cooper, D. R.; Terman, D. S.; Marck, R.: Ex vivo removal of serum-IgG in a patient with colon carcinoma: Biochemical, immunological, and histological observations. Cancer *42;* 1 (1979).
3   Frosgren, A.; Sjöquist, J.: Protein-A from S. aureus I pseudoimmune reaction with human γ-globulin. J. Immun. *97:* 822 (1966).
4   Glöckner, W. M.; Sieberth, H. G.: Plasmafiltration: A new method of plasma exchange. Proc. Europ. Soc. artif. Organs *5:* 214 (1978).
5   Israel, L.; Samak, R.; Edelstein, R.: Multiple plasma-exchange therapy for metastatic cancer. In: Sieberth (ed.), Plasma Exchange, p. 381 (F. K. Schattauer Verlag, Stuttgart, New York 1980).

6 Kessler, S. W.: Rapid isolation of antigens from cells with a staphylococcal protein-A-antibody adsorbent; Parameters of the interaction of antibody-antigen complexes with protein-A. J. Immun. *115:* 1617 (1975).

7 Lupien, P. J.; Moorjani, S.; Lou, M.; Brun, D.; Gagni, C.: Removal of cholesterol from blood by affinity binding to heparin-agarose: Evaluation on treatment in homocygous familial hypercholesterolemia. Pediat. Res. *14:* 113 (1980).

8 Malchesky, P. S.; Asanuma, Y.; Zawicki, I.; Blumenstein, M.; Calabrese, L.; Kyo, A.; Krankauer, R.; Nosé, Y.: On line separation of macromolecules by membrane filtration with cryogelation. In: Sieberth (ed.), Plasma Exchange, p. 133 (F. K. Schattauer Verlag, Stuttgart–New York 1980).

9 Price, P. B.; Walker, R. U.: Chemical etching of charged particles cracked in solids. J. appl. Physics *33:* 3406 (1962).

10 Ray, P. K.: Immunoadsorption of IgG molecules from the plasma. Jahrestagung der Arbeitsgemeinschaft für klinische Nephrologie, Würzburg 1980 (in press).

11 Scharschmidt, B. F.; Martin, J. F.; Shapiro, L. J.; Platz, P. H.; Berk, P. D.: Hemoperfusion through albumin-conjugated agarose gel for the treatment of neonatal jaundice in premature rhesus monkeys. J. Lab. clin. Med. *89:* 101 (1977).

12 Solomon, B. A.; Costino, F.; Lysaght, M. J.; Colton, C. K.; Friedmann, L. C.: Continuous-flow membrane filtration of plasma from whole blood. Trans. Am. Soc. artif. internal Organs *24:* 21 (1978).

13 Sieberth, H. G.: The elimination of defined substances from the blood and from separated plasma. In: Sieberth (ed.), Plasma Exchange, p. 29 (F. K. Schattauer Verlag, Stuttgart–New York 1980).

14 Stoffel, W.; Demant, Th.; Sieberth, H. G.; Borberg, H.; Glöckner, W. M.: Selective removal of Apo-B containing serum lipoproteins from blood plasma. In: Sieberth (ed.), Plasma Exchange, p. 127 (F. K. Schattauer Verlag, Stuttgart–New York 1980).

15 Terman, D. S.; Yamamoto, T.; Mattioli, M.; Cook, G.; Tillquist, R.; Henry, J.; Poser, R.; Daskal, Y.: Extension necrosis of spontaneous canine mammary adenocarcinoma after extracorporeal perfusion over Staphylococcus aureus Cowan I. 1. Description of acute tumoricidal response: Morphologic, histologic, immunohistochemical, immunologic, and serological bindings. J. Immun. *124:* 795 (1980).

Prof. Dr. H.-G. Sieberth, Abt. Innere Medizin II, Rhein.-Westf. Technische Hochschule Aachen, Goethestr. 27–29, D-5100 Aachen

Double Filtration Plasmapheresis and Immunoadsorption: Technical Aspect

Tetsuzo Agishi

Kidney Center, Tokyo Women's Medical College, Tokyo, Japan

A new technique for plasmapheresis has been developed in an attempt to eliminate disadvantages from conventional plasmapheresis, namely, the necessity for an expensive centrifuge and human blood products.

The new method, named double filtration plasmapheresis, utilizes two filters with different pore sizes, one of which separates plasma from whole blood during extracorporeal circulation, and another filtrates smaller molecular components from the filtrated plasma. The filtrate of the second filter is then mixed with the formed blood elements and returned to patient. Consequently, larger molecular plasma components are supposed to be selectively removed and only need to be replaced with 500–600 ml of human blood product or synthetic plasma expander. Over 120 preliminary clinical applications have been performed in 22 patients mainly with immunologic diseases and peripheral circulatory disorders.

Clinically satisfactory effects have been observed in almost all patients. However, selective removal of larger molecular components of plasma has not been satisfactorily achieved and a certain amount of albumin fraction is proved to leak out of the system.

Removal of the immunologic substances by extracorporeal adsorption offers the possibility for stricter selectivity. Adsorption capability of more than 20 synthetic materials has been investigated by measuring gamma globulin and immunoelectrophoresis.

Some of porous inorganics are more suitable and interesting for this purpose.

I. Double Filtration Plasmapheresis

I.1. Introduction

Plasmapheresis is expected to offer a possibility for a new treatment of immunologic diseases, hyperviscosity syndrome, and extensive cancer.

Plasmapheresis is one of the blood purification procedures and very similar to hemodialysis, hemocarboperfusion, or hemofiltration in terms of the technical aspects of extracorporeal circulation, but different from them in terms of the substances aimed to be removed.

As plasmapheresis is a new technique, its clinical application has not yet been firmly established and some problems can be pointed out in actual performance.

Although a continuous centrifuge has been traditionally used in standard plasmapheresis, the recent development in modern membrane technology enables plasma to be separated from whole blood by filtration [1].

Necessity for an expensive centifuge and voluminous human blood products for substitution in existing plasmapheresis modalities prove to be problematic for a popular application of this treatment.

Double filtration plasmapheresis is devised to solve the problems mentioned above [2].

I.2. Principle of Double Filtration Plasmapheresis

A basic principle of double filtration plasmapheresis is to consecutively filtrate blood components by using two filters with different pore sizes (fig. 1). Filter with larger pores separates plasma directly from cell-rich whole blood during extracorporeal circulation and is led into another filter with smaller pores. Smaller molecular fraction of plasma is filtrated, mixed with cell-rich whole blood, and returned to patient. Larger molecular fraction of plasma is theoretically concentrated during the procedure and discarded.

Double filtration plasmapheresis aims to remove the relatively larger molecular fractions, such as antibodies or immunecomplexes, while leaving smaller molecular fractions than albumin in the blood.

I.3. Property of Filters

The first filter, the plasma separator, is composed of hollow fibers made of polyvinyl-alcohol membrane with an average pore size of 0.4 micron. A scan electron microscope reveals a sponge-like structure of this

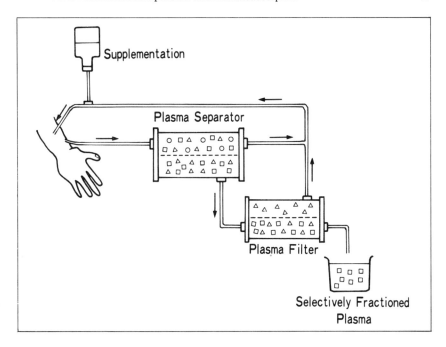

Fig. 1. Principle of double filtration plasmapheresis.

material. 1,000 ml/h plasma is easily obtained by the plasma separator at natural flow resistance of lower than 50 mm Hg.

The second filter, plasma filter, is an ethylene-vinyl-alcohol hollow-fiber membrane with pores of approximately 0.1 micron. Filtration rate is controlled by adjusting filtration pressure with a screw cramp on an outlet line.

In vitro examinations, using various molecular weight of dextran, suggest that approximately 70% of albumin (69,000 dalton) can be retrieved while approximately 95% of immunoglobulins (approximately 200,000 dalton) can be removed from the whole system, if these solutes are transferred in a very similar manner as dextran.

I.4. Clinical Performance

As usual, 2,500 to 3,000 ml of plasma is separated by the plasma separator in 2½ to 3 h. 500 to 600 ml of concentrated larger molecular fractions of plasma is produced and replaced with 6% HES (hydroxyethyl starch) or 5% human albumin in lactated Ringer's solution.

By the end of October 1980, 126 double filtration plasmaphereses have been performed on 22 patients with immunologic diseases such as SLE, PSS, renal transplantation and MG, circulatory disturbances such as Buerger's diseases and arteriosclerosis, and extensive carcinoma.

Various clinical effects depend upon the original disease and have been reported elsewhere [3, 4].

Only technical aspects of performance of double filtration plasmapheresis will be discussed in this report.

(a) Hemodynamics during double filtration plasmapheresis.

No noticeable changes are present in blood pressure and pulse rate during double filtration plasmapheresis while substituting with albumin and HES.

(b) Hematology during double filtration plasmapheresis.

Almost no marked changes in red blood-cell count, hematocrit, and platelet count are observed after double filtration plasmapheresis. Only a slight increase in white blood-cell count is observed in both albumin and HES replacement. This phenomenon is probably similar to that observed in hemodialysis, but its clinical significance remains unknown.

(c) Filtration coefficient for various substances.

Filtration coefficient for plasma separator is defined as the concentration of the particular substance in filtrate of the plasma separator, divided by the concentration of the substance in the blood coming into the whole system (fig. 2).

The coefficient is very close to 1.0 for small molecular substances. However, there is a tendency that as molecular weight increases the coefficient becomes smaller though there are some exceptions. The coefficient for hemoglobin is extremely large. This is explained by hemolysis on the plasmaseparator membrane surface on special occasions with high filtration pressure. Hemoglobin, which usually does not exist in blood coming into the system, easily passes through the membrane of the plasma separator.

Concentration coefficient for plasma filter is defined as the concentration of the particular substance in plasma fraction to be discarded, divided by the concentration of the substance in the filtrate of the plasma separator.

The coefficient is again very close to 1.0 for the small molecular

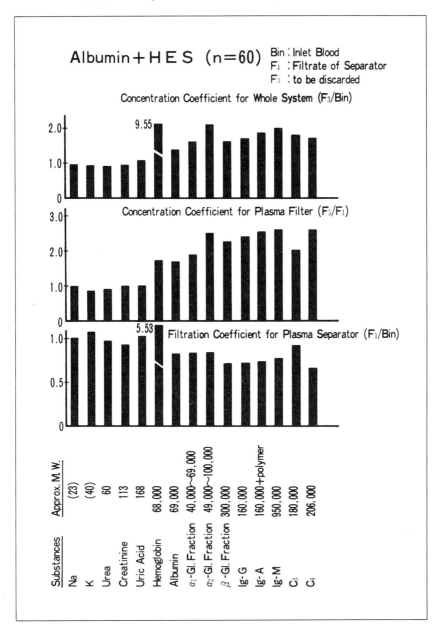

Fig. 2. Coefficients for various substances.

substances, and increases as molecular weight of the substances increases as a result of the large molecular substances' inability to pass through the plasma filter.

Concentration coefficient for whole system is defined as the concentration of the particular substance in plasma fraction to be discarded, divided by the concentration of the substance in the blood coming into the system.

The coefficient is once again very close to 1.0 for molecular substances smaller than uric acid in this evaluation. This means that small molecular substances do not concentrate in the system. However, the coefficient increases for the substances with larger molecular weights. This proves that large molecular substances are selectively concentrated in double filtration plasmapheresis. An important observation is that the coefficient for albumin is slightly larger than 1.0, even though it is smaller than those for globulin fractions, C3 and C4. A certain amount of albumin is concentrated by the system and discarded.

Comparative evaluation in concentration coefficient is conducted between albumin and HES supplementation (fig. 3).

Filtration coefficient for plasma separator is approximately 0.8 for

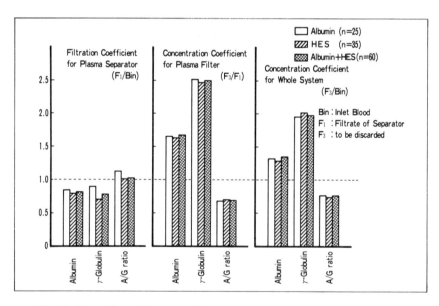

Fig. 3. Comparison of concentration coefficients between albumin and HES supplementations.

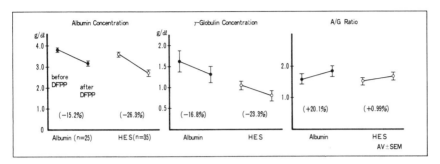

Fig. 4. Comparison of plasma protein concentrations in albumin and HES supplementations.

albumin and gamma globulin both in albumin and HES supplementation. Subsequently, A/G ratio is approximately 1.0.

Concentration coefficient for plasma filter for albumin is much smaller than for gamma globulin both in albumin and HES supplementation.

Concentration coefficient for the whole system for albumin is approximately 1.3, and much smaller than 2.1 for gamma globulin both in albumin and HES supplementation.

There is no difference in the concentration between supplementation with albumin and HES.

Effect of double filtration plasmapheresis on plasma-protein concentration is compared between albumin and HES supplementation. Average albumin concentration is lower in HES than albumin supplementation after double filtration plasmapheresis. A very similar effect is observed in gamma globulin concentration. It is hard to explain the latter (fig. 4).

Removal of immunoglobulins is assessed and graphically depicted. There is a high concentration in immunoglobulins before plasmapheresis. A considerable amount of immunoglobulins is removed from the system both in albumin and HES supplementation. However, a quatitative comparison is not made because of insufficient data.

1.5. Comment

Considerable selective concentration and removal of large molecular fractions of plasma such as immunoglobulins and complements are possible with the current double filtration plasmapheresis technique utilizing presently available filters as evidenced by laboratory data and clinical improvements in symptoms [3, 4]. However, the problem still exists that a certain amount of albumin is also removed by the current system. Leakage of albumin is due to the insufficient filtration ability of the plasma filter. Development of such filter material which sharply cuts off albumin is urgent.

II. Immunoadsorption

II.1. Introduction

Extracorporeal removal of immunologic substances by adsorption is expected to offer stricter selectivity. Experimental specific removal of antigen or antibody with immobilized corresponding antibody or antigen has already been reported [5]. Advantage of this method is its extremely keen selectivity in removing the aimed substance. However, disadvantages are first its instability, caused by the removal of target substance as biological process is involved, and, secondly, difficulty in procuring a sufficient amount of antigen or antibody for column assembly.

It has been well recognized that protein fraction of blood adheres to

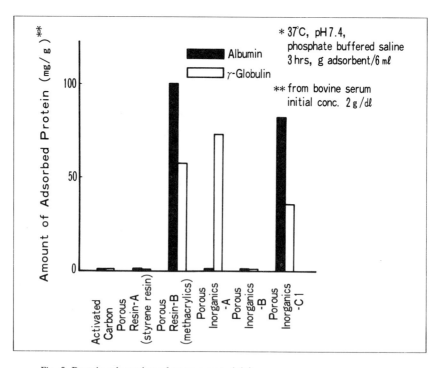

Fig. 5. Protein adsorption of porous materials*.

the surface of foreign materials, and component patterns of adsorbed proteins are specific for each material.

Materials consisting of polymers and inorganics have been screened in an attempt to find suitable immunoadsorbents which selectively adsorb immunologic substances.

II.2. Adsorbents for Plasma Protein

Although activated charcoal, porous resin A of polystyrene type and porous inorganic B do not adsorb plasma protein, porous resin B of methacrylate type, porous inorganic A and C-1 adsorb proteins well in in vitro batch study using bovine albumin and gamma globulin (fig. 5). Especially porous inorganic A shows selective adsorbability of gamma globulin.

As albumin is an acidotic protein and gamma globulin is a neutral or basic protein, electric charge on material surface is anticipated to present some effect on the selectiveness in adsorbability. Therefore, negative charge is introduced either by surface coating or chemical treatment of the surface in order to improve selectivity to gamma globulin adsorption.

Porous resin B shows reduced albumin adsorption and increased

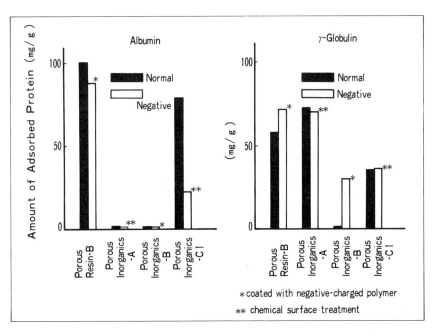

Fig. 6. Effect of surface negativity of porous materials on protein adsorption.

gamma globulin adsorption after acidification of the surface (fig. 6). Porous inorganic B shows gamma globulin adsorbability after the treatment in spite of almost no adsorption of proteins before the treatment. There is no effect from acidification of porous inorganic A. In porous inorganic C-1, albumin adsorption is markedly reduced while gamma globulin adsorption is unaltered. As a result, selectivity in gamma globulin adsorbability is improved. In vitro evaluation utilizing porous inorganic C-4 shows that 90 % of gamma globulin is removed from the plasma of a SLE patient while only 10 % of albumin is reduced.

Subsequently, animal experiment is performed with rabbits. Blood of rabbits is perfused through a porous inorganic C-4 column via extracorporeal circulation. Gamma globulin level reduces to 20 % of the initial level 1 h after beginning the perfusion. Albumin level reduces to 80 % of the initial level after 1 h and does not show any change thereafter.

II.3. Comment

It has been shown that some of porous inorganics selectively adsorb plasma gamma globulin, and there is the possibility to improve selectivity by means of physiochemical modification of the material surface. Adsorbents such as described here are expected to be useful as immunoadsorbents in treatment of immunologic diseases by removing immunologic substances during extracorporeal circulation.

References

1   Solomon, B. A.; Castino, F.; Lysaght, M. J.; Colton, D. K.; Friedman, L. I.: Continuous-flow membrane filtration of plasma from whole blood. Trans. ASAIO 24: 21–26 (1978).
2   Agishi, T.; Kaneko, I.; Hasuo, Y.; Kumagaya, E.; Hayasaka, Y; Ota, K.; Sugino, N.; Abe, M.; Ono, T.; Kawai, S.; Yamane, T.: Double filtration for selective removal or retrieval of plasma fraction. ASAIO (Abstracts) 8: 70 (1979).
3   Agishi, T.; Kaneko, I.; Hasuo, Y.; Hayasaka, Y.; Sanaka, T.; Ota, K.; Abe, M.; Ono, T.; Kawai, S.; Yamane, K.: Double filtration plasmapheresis. Trans. Am. Soc. artif. internal Organs 26: 406–411 (1980).
4   Agishi, T.; Kaneko, I.; Hasuo, Y.; Hayasaka, Y.; Sanaka, T.; Ota, K.; Amemiya, H.; Sugino, N.: Double filtration plasmapheresis with no or minimal amount of blood derivatives for substituion. In: Sieberth (ed.), Plasma exchange, pp. 53–57 (F. K. Schattauer Verlag, Stuttgart-New York 1980).
5   Terman, D. S.; Stewart, I.: Specific removal of circulating antigen by means of immunoadsorption. FEBS Lett. 61 (1): 59–62 (1976).

Tetsuzo Agishi, MD, Professor, Kidney Center, Tokyo Women's Medical College, 10 Kawada-cho, Shinjuku-ku, Tokyo 162, Japan

Plasma Removal Using the Fenwal® Membrane Plasmapheresis System

D. H. Buchholz, Cynthia Helphingstine, Judith Houx Porten

Fenwal Laboratories, Division of Travenol Laboratories, Inc., Deerfield, Ill./USA

Although the harvest of donor plasma using techniques in which erythrocytes were returned to the donor was described in the early 1900s, for many years most plasma utilized for transfusion or fractionation purposes was derived as a byproduct from the donation of whole blood. Since the frequency of whole-blood donation is limited by the time required for erythrocyte regeneration, only relatively small amounts of plasma can be collected yearly from any one whole-blood donor. While plasmapheresis techniques were utilized to a limited extent in the 1950s as was the Cohn fractionator, it was not until the advent of disposable plastic blood-collection systems that selective and repeated plasma harvest from the same donor became feasible.

In addition to the use of whole-blood collection and plasmapheresis techniques in harvesting plasma for transfusion or fractionation, plasma-exchange transfusion is playing an increasingly important role in the management of a number of immunologically mediated diseases. Although exchange can be performed by manual (Blood Pack®) techniques, more rapid exchange is possible by using a variety of semi-automated instruments including the NCI-IBM 2990-6 Experimental Blood-Cell Separator, the Haemonetics Model 30™ Blood Processor, the IBM 2997™ Blood-Cell Separator, the Celltrifuge® Blood-Cell Separator, and the Fenwal CS-3000® Blood-Cell Separator. By using these instruments, it has become possible to return patient erythrocytes while discarding autologous plasma (which presumably contains 'unwanted' materials or lacks 'normal' substances) and replacing it with albumin, saline, plasma-protein fraction or fresh-frozen single donor plasma.

The above instruments use a variety of differently shaped centrifuge bowls to separate plasma from erythrocytes; all, however, require the use of centrifugal force to effect the separation. Recently Fenwal Laboratories, Division of Travenol Laboratories, Inc. has developed a cross-flow filtration system patterned after a device developed by *Friedman et al.* [1] and studied by *Wiltbank et al.* [2, 3] which permits cell-free plasma to be removed from whole blood without the need for centrifugation. To achieve plasma separation, blood is passed at high shear rates between a folded sheet of microporous membrane (400 cm^2). The membrane is housed in a filtration cell similar to that shown schematically in figure 1. The cell consists of two outer rigid covers (C, fig. 1) which are bolted together and two inner flexible plates (B) which support the membrane (A) and provide channels for the removal of collected plasma. Whole blood enters at one end of the filtration cell (F), passes between the folded membrane, and exits from the opposite end (D). Platelets, leukocytes, and erythrocytes are retained by the membrane while plasma passes through small ($\simeq$ 0.6 micron diameter) pores and is channeled by the membrane-support plates to one end of the cell where it is removed (E).

To achieve the shear rates needed for efficient plasma separation ($\simeq$ 2000/s), a portion of the processed blood is recirculated through the filtration cell at approximately 200 ml/min. Use of a recirculation loop permits plasma removal at rates of 17 to 23 ml/min from donors/patients with normal hematocrits without the need for arterio-venous fistulae or shunts to obtain high blood-withdrawal rates. By using this device, blood is typically withdrawn at 50–70 ml/min and pumped through the filtration cell; a portion of blood is then recirculated while the remainder is returned via a second vein. Plasma flux varies with the rate of blood withdrawal, the intermembrane distance, the transmembrane pressure, and the donor/patient hematocrit.

The filtration cell is used in conjunction with an instrument console, similar to that shown in figure 2. The console contains three peristaltic pumps used for blood withdrawal, anticoagulant administration (anticoagulant citrate dextrose (ACD), formula-A, mixed with blood in a ratio of 1:8 to 1:15 parts of ACD to blood), and blood recirculation through the cell. A sensitive electronic scale monitors the weight of plasma removed and instrument display indicators show blood-withdrawal rate, blood-recirculation rate, plasma-removal rate, anticoagulant-flow rate, membrane pressure, the volume of blood processed, and the volume of plasma removed. The instrument is equipped with a number of donor/patient safety monitors do detect occluded blood withdrawal or return lines, to

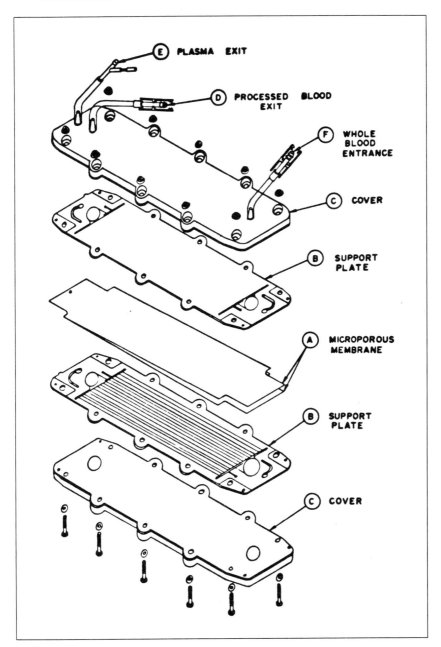

Fig. 1. Exploded view schematic of prototype cross-flow filtration cell used for membrane plasmapheresis.

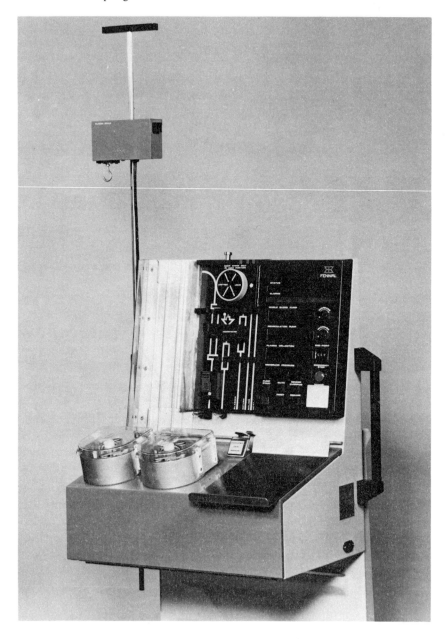

Fig. 2. Prototype instrument console used for blood processing in conjunction with the cross-flow filtration cell. The cell is inserted in a clamp at the left edge of the console panel. The anticoagulant pump is not shown in this figure.

sense excessive membrane pressure, to detect hemolysis in collected plasma, and to detect and trap air or foam which may enter the blood-processing pathway. In addition, there is a sensor which alerts the operator if the anticoagulant container becomes empty. These safety monitors function in such a way as to both alert the operator of abnormal operating conditions and automatically stop the blood-processing procedure.

The membrane plasmapheresis cell and instrument console currently are being evaluated in the United States in the laboratories of William Bayer, MD, Kansas City, Missouri; Jacob Nusbacher, MD, Rochester, New York; and Aaron Josephson, MD, Chicago, Illinois. Although the device was designed to perform plasma-exchange transfusions, initial clinical evaluations have been directed at plasma collection in normal donors in order to establish instrument safety and efficacy. In these studies, 550 ml of plasma was harvested during a 30–40 min collection period and compared with pre- and post-collection donor plasma using various chemical, coagulation, and hematologic assays. It should be noted that collected plasma is slightly diluted compared with pre- and post-donation plasma due to the presence of anticoagulant citrate dextrose and to a small amount of saline which remains in the plasma line and collection bag following the priming process.

A total of 46 collections has been performed using this system. Donor hematologic and coagulation profile changes before and after removal of 550 ml of plasma are shown in table I. While there were no significant changes in donor hematocrit, platelet count, prothrombin time, partial thromboplastin time, fibrinogen, or plasma hemoglobin, there was a slight decline in the donor leukocyte and granulocyte count at the completion of the collection. Coagulation factor V, VII, and IX activity in post-donation and collected plasma was slightly diminished consistent with hemodilution. Factor VIII activity showed a large drop from an unexpectedly high value of 186 U/dl prior to donation to a more normal mean value of 104 by the completion of the procedure; activity in collected plasma averaged 134 U/dl. The high mean pre-procedure value of 186 U/dl may have resulted from epinephrine release consequent to donor apprehension regarding blood donation using "a new experimental device," with a return to normal values as the procedure progressed. There was no evidence of platelet aggregation or blood clotting within the blood-processing pathway in any of the 46 procedures. The collected plasma contained a mean of 0.06×10^6 red blood cells/µl and 4×10^3 platelets/µl; no

Table I. Hematologic and coagulation profile changes associated with membrane plasmapheresis

	No. procedures	Donor pre-collection	Donor post-collection	Collected plasma*
Hematocrit (vol/dl)	46	42	42	$RBC = 0.06 \times 10^6/\mu l$
Platelet count (x10³/μl)	46	242	227	4
WBC count (x10³/μl)	46	6.4	4.8	0
PMN count (x10³/μl)	41	3.7	3.0	0
Prothrombin time (s)	34	11.9	12.4	13.1
Partial thromboplastin time (s)	34	39	42	42
Fibrinogen (mg/dl)	34	210	196	185
Factor V (U/dl)	11	113	82	84
Factor VII (U/dl)	11	116	87	96
Factor VIII (U/dl)	11	186	104	134
Factor IX (U/dl)	11	155	126	135

* Collected plasma slightly diluted by saline prime solution and by anticoagulant relative to pre-collection values

leukocytes were seen. Coagulation-factor activity was similar to that seen in the donor immediately following the completion of the procedure.

Changes in blood chemical parameters are shown in table II. There was no evidence of red blood-cell lysis or damage as indicated by normal plasma hemoglobin values, nor were there medically significant unexpected changes in other donor-blood chemistries. The elevated glucose and reduced calcium values seen in collected plasma likely reflect the presence of the ACD used for anticoagulation. It is of interest to note that large molecules, such as IgM and factor VIII appear to traverse the microporous membrane with ease.

All donors tolerated the plasma-collection procedure without difficulty although one noted slight perioral tingling and 7 others felt chilly. Although extracorporeal blood volume is small ($\simeq$ 150 ml), use of a blood warmer likely will be required during therapeutic exchange transfusion since significant heat loss will likely occur from the tubing and filtration cell during the course of an exchange transfusion.

It should be emphasized that the filtration cell and prototype instrument console have been developed primarily for use in therapeutic plasma-exchange procedures. The testing described in this report was performed with normal donors to permit quantification of hematological, chemical, and coagulation changes associated with the blood-processing

Table II. Blood chemical profile changes associated with membrane plasmapheresis

	No. procedures	Donor pre-collection	Donor post-collection	Collected plasma*
Plasma hemoglobin (mg/dl)		1	1	3
Glucose (mg/dl)	38	99	97	313
Blood urea nitrogen (mg/dl)	37	13	12	8
Creatinine (mg/dl)	38	1.0	0.9	0.8
Calcium (mg/dl)	37	9.0	8.6	4.9
Inorganic phosphorus (mg/dl)	38	3.6	3.0	2.6
Total bilirubin (mg/dl)	38	0.5	0.5	0.3
Lactate dehydrogenase (U/1)	38	133	119	101
Glutamic oxaloacetic transaminase (U/1)	36	24	23	19
Alkaline phosphatase (U/1)	37	60	50	42
Uric acid (mg/dl)	38	5.5	5.2	4.1
Cholesterol (mg/dl)	38	182	161	131
Total protein (g/dl)	38	6.6	5.9	5.1
Albumin (g/dl)	38	4.4	3.9	3.3
IgG (mg/dl)	23	776	667	673
IgA (mg/dl)	23	185	149	162
IgM (mg/dl)	23	107	87	92

* Collected plasma slightly diluted by saline prime solution and by anticoagulant relative to pre-collection values

procedure. These studies could not be performed in patients undergoing exchange transfusion since post-donation measurements would reflect only the composition of the fluid being returned to the patient and likely would not permit detection of subtle changes associated with use of the cross-flow filtration system. Plasma-exchange studies are currently underway in the United States; preliminary studies show no decline in membrane performance during the time necessary for 3–4 l exchanges. As expected, plasma-removal rates are inversely proportional to the patient's hematocrit. In one patient with a hematocrit of 20 vol/dl, plasma has been collected at a flow rate of 40 ml/min throughout a 3 l exchange procedure.

The above studies demonstrate the usefulness of the membrane plasmapheresis concept for plasma separation using a completely disposable blood-processing pathway that does not require the use of centrifugal force. Continuous-flow processing at low blood-withdrawal rates permits rapid plasma removal without the need for fistulae or shunts, thus avoiding the need for a surgical procedure in the recipient being exchanged. The collected plasma is not hemolyzed, contains only very small numbers of red blood cells and platelets, and appears to be of similar composition to that of the patient, with large molecules easily passing through the membrane. Although plasma-exchange trials are not yet complete, initial observations suggest that this easily mobile system will be very useful in performing therapeutic exchange procedures.

References

1 Friedman, L. I.; Castino, F.; Lysaght, M. J.; Solomon, B. A.; Sanderson, J. E.; Wiltbank, T. B.: A continuous-flow plasmapheresis system. Final Report: National Heart, Lung and Blood Institute (USA) Contract No. 1–HB–6–2928 (June 1976 to April 1979).
2 Wiltbank, T. B.; Castino, F.; Grapka, B.; Friedman, L. I.; Solomon, B. A.: Filtration plasmapheresis – initial in vivo studies. Transfusion *18:* 627 (1978).
3 Wiltbank, T. B.; Castino, F.; Grapka, B.; Daniels, J.; Friedman, L. I.: Filtration plasmapheresis – donor evaluation studies. Transfusion *19:* 666 (1979).

D. H. Buchholz, MD, Fenwal Laboratories, USA–Deerfield, Ill. 60015

Clinical Tolerance and Hazards of Plasma Exchanges: A Study of 6200 Plasma Exchanges in 1033 Patients*

J. P. Aufeuvre[2], F. Mortin-Hertel[1], M. Cohen-Solal[1], A. Lefloch[1], J. Baudelot[1]

[1] Centre Departemental de Transfusion Sanguine, Hopital Avicenne, Bobigny, France
[2] Centre Departemental de Transfusion Sanguine, Yvelines-Nord, Poissy, France

Plasma exchange (PE) is a new therapeutic procedure which has undergone considerable development during recent years.

The biological consequences of repeated PE have been extensively investigated [2, 3, 6, 7, 9, 10]. This, however, has not been the case for their clinical tolerance [1, 4, 5, 11].

* With the collaboration of the following centers:

C.R.T.S. – 06	St. Laurent du Var	Dr. R. Follana
C.R.T.S. – 31	Toulouse	Dr. J. Ducos
C.D.T.S. – 38	Grenoble	Dr. F. Chenais
C.D.T.S. – 42	St. Etienne	Dr. B. Gannat
C.D.T.S. – 51	Reims	Dr. J. C. Adjizian
C.D.T.S. – 63	Clermont Ferrand	Dr. J. M. Bidet
C.R.T.S. – 69	Lyon	Dr. P. Tremisi
C.R.T.S. – 67	Strasbourg	Dr. C. Waller
C.D.T.S. – 74	Annemasse	Dr. N. Coudurier
C.H.P. – 75	Paris Hop. St. Antoine	Dr. Y. Brossart
C.T.S. – 75	Paris Hop. Pitie-Salp.	Dr. S. Theirry
C.T.S. – 75	Paris Hop. St. Louis	Dr. A. Bussel
C.R.T.S. – 76	Bois Guillaume	Dr. J. C. Bonneau
C.D.T.S. – 86	Poitiers	Dr. D. Alcalay
C.D.T.S. – 93	Bobigny	Dr. J. P. Aufeuvre
C.D.T.S. – 94	Creteil	Dr. E. Radeau
C.D.T.S. – 95	Pontoise	Dr. F. Grosdhomme
C.H.U. –	Dijon	Dr. G. Rifle
C.R.L.C. –	Montpellier	Dr. B. Serrou
C.D.T.S. – 74	Annecy	Dr. R. Gotteland

In order to appreciate the clinical tolerance of this method, we sent a questionnaire in July 1979 (table I) to each French institute performing PEs. A year later, in September 1980, we sent another questionnaire to the teams who participated in the first study. The second study was restricted to serious accidents.

Results

The first study (1979) allowed us to collect 3,431 PEs performed in 592 patients by 19 teams (table II). Several cases were not evaluable. The statistics were derived from 3,086 PEs in 512 patients.

The various indications of PE and their respective frequencies are calculated from the 399 diagnoses made in 512 patients (tables III and IV).

22% of PE are disturbed by one or more clinical incidents (table V). We only considered the immediate side effects.

Table I. Questionnaire (1979)

	CFC*	IFC**
1 *Number of patients treated*		
2 *Diagnosis*		
3 *Number of exchanges*		
4 *Replacement solution used*		
5 *Number of minor incidents*		
(symp. of hypocalcemia – nausea – vomiting – urticaria)		
a) Leading to drug administration		
b) Leading to interruption of the exchange		
6 *Number of chills – hyperthermia syndromes*		
a) as above		
b) as above		
7 *Number of serious accidents leading to*		
more important therapeutic acts		
Give a brief report of such cases.		
8 *In which medical surrounding are you working*		
– Blood bank within the hospital	YES	NO
– Direct connection with the resuscitation unit	YES	NO
9 *Have you some comments* to make about this questionarre or the clinical tolerance of plasma exchanges?		

* continous-flow centrifugation
** intermittent-flow centrifugation

Table II. First questionnaire (1979)

	Number of teams	Number of patients	Number of PE	Mean number of PE/patient
CFC	7	100	546	5.4
IFC	14	412	2540	6.1
Total	19*	592**	3431***	6

* Two teams used either CFC or IFC
** Some answers are not detailed enough and 80 patients cannot be classified
*** For the same reasons some PE cannot be classified

Table III. Indications of PE (399 diagnosis known out of 592 patients) 1979

Solid tumors	99	I.T.P.	3
Dysglobulinemias	90	Rheumatoid arthritis	3
Auto-imm. diseases	42	Intoxications	2
Myasthenia gravis	29	Non-obstructive cardio-myopathy	
Connective tissue dis.	26	Hyperthyroids	
Allo. anti-D	22	Henoch-Schönlein purpura	
G. nephritis	17	Porphyria	
Incompatible ABO Ab	13	Endotoxic shock	
Renal-transplant rejection	12	Fulminant hepatitis	
Non-myelomatous dysproteinemias	7	Necrosing vasculitis	1
Leukemias	6	Cardiac-transplant rejection	
Correction of bleeding time	4	Sphingo-lipidosis	
Anti-F. VIII Ab	4	Pemphigus	
Goodpasture's syndrome	4	Fulminant purpura	
Cryoglobulinemias	3	Behcet's disease	
		Nephro-anemic syndrome	

Table IV. The most frequent indications (81.2% of PE) 1979

Diagnosis	No. of patients	% of plasma exchanges						
Solid tumors	99	24.8	–	–	–	–	–	–
Dysglobulinemias	90	22.5	47.3	–	–	–	–	–
Auto-immu. disease	42	10.5	–	57.8	–	–	–	–
Myasthenia gravis	29	7.2	–	–	65	–	–	–
Connective-tissue. disease	26	6.5	–	–	–	71.5	–	–
Allo anti.D Ab	22	5.5	–	–	–	–	77	–
G. nephritis	17	4.2	–	–	–	–	–	81.2

Table V. PEs are disturbed by one or more clinical incidents (1979)

	Minor incidents			Chills/hyperthermia			Serious accidents	Total
	N	Drugs	Stop	N	Drugs	Stop	N	N
CFC (n = 546)	108	96	2	81	71	0	8	675
IFC (n = 2450)	382	243	30	85	61	8	11	(22%)
Total 3086								

We divided the side effects into 3 groups:

(1) Minor incidents such as urticaria, hypocalcemia, gastro-intestinal manifestations, transient drop in blood pressure are the most frequent causes and disturb 15.8% of PEs (fig. 1). Most of them (70%) lead to drug administration, mainly corticosteroids, antihistamics, and calcium gluconate. In very few cases, PE must be stopped (1%) owing to the severity of these manifestations.

(2) Chills and hyperthermia are less frequent and only occur in 5.3% of PEs. Almost all of them (93%) require drug administration but seldom lead to the interruption of the exchange (fig. 1).

(3) Serious accidents do not answer to any accurate definition; the classification as a serious accident was made by those performing PEs. Their number and frequency are calculated from the answers to the first and second questionnaires. The latter only dealt with those serious accidents which occurred since the first study. We only received 11 answers out of 19 teams who participated in the first study (2,769 plasma exchanges in 441 patients).

6,200 plasma exchanges performed in 1,033 patients were complicated by 33 serious accidents (table VI), of which 7 patients died.

The pulmonary and cardiovascular complications were the most frequent causes for these accidents (table VII) and were observed in the 7 deaths appearing in this study (table VIII).

Case 1

A young pregnant woman with a high titer of allo-anti-D. experienced chills and cyanosis after 1.51 of plasma had been exchanged (this was not her first PE) followed by a rough cough preceding an acute

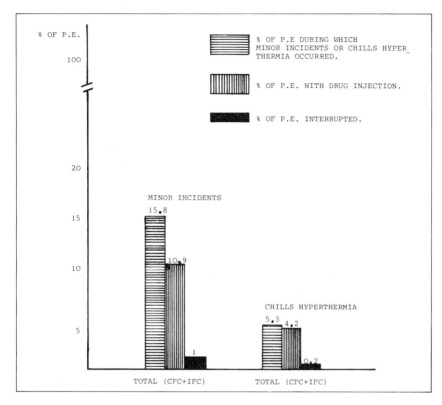

Fig. 1. Incidence of minor incidents and chills/hyperthermia syndromes (3086 PE), 1979.

pulmonary edema which did not respond to therapy. The patient died during the night.

This pulmonary edema did not seem to be of hemodynamic origin. Antileukocyte antibodies (not anti-HLA) were presumed to be responsible, but this has not yet been proven.

Case 2

A 56-year-old woman suffering from rheumatoid arthritis developed, during the 5th exchange, an acute pulmonary edema, similar to the preceding case, with cough and dyspnea which could not be related to a volume imbalance. The patient died during the night.

Table VI. Serious accidents complicated PEs (1979 + 1980)

	CFC	IFC	Total
Number of patients	133	810	1033*
Number of PE	758	5097	6200**
Number of accidents	11	22	33
Mean number of PE/patient	5.6	6.2	6

* Some answers are not detailed enough and 90 patients cannot be classified
** For the same reasons some PE cannot be classified

Table VII. Causes of accidents (1979 + 1980)

		Total	%
Pulmonary accidents			
Pulmonary edema	13		
Acute pulmonary failure	2	16	48.5
Massive pulmonary embolism	1		
Cardiovascular accidents			
Cardiovascular collapses	4		
Angor	2		
Cardio-pulmonary failure	1	12	36.4
Paroxysmal hypertension	1		
Cerebral spasm in H. T. patient	1		
Paroxysmal cardiac dysrhythmias	3		
Diverse			
Epilepsia	1		
Quincke's edema	1		
Anaphylactic shock	1	5	15.1
Metabolic alkalosis	1		
D.I.C.	1		
Total		33	

Table VIII. 7 deaths out of 1033 patients during 6200 exchanges (1979 + 1980)

Non-hemodynamic acute pulmonary edema	2
Paroxysmal cardiac dysrhythmias	3
Hemodynamic acute pulmonary edema	1
Massive pulmonary embolism	1

The pathologist's conclusion was a lesional pulmonary edema. In these 2 cases, fresh-frozen plasma (FFP) was used as a replacement solution.

Case 3

A 69-year-old woman suffered from cirrhosis, portal hypertension, monoclonal IgM, and peripheral neuropathy due to vasculitis. During the 9th exchange, she had dyspnea and tachycardia, a convulsive crisis, and finally cardiac arrest. She was resuscitated, but remained in a deep coma and died during the night.

The necropsy did not reveal the cause of death and a paroxysmal dysrhythmia was presumed to be responsible.

Case 4

A 54-year-old woman had chronic lymphocytic leukemia and monoclonal IgM. She had had plasma exchanges for more than 1 year with very good results. At the very end of an exchange, she had cardiac arrest and could not be resuscitated.

The necropsy did not reveal the cause of death as in the preceding case. The coronary arteries were normal; there was no pulmonary embolism; nor edema; but her myocardial septum was infiltrated by lymphoid tissue and we supposed that this could have facilitated the occurrence of a paroxysmal cardiac dysrhythmia.

Case 5

A 45-year-old woman had IgA gammapathy with very rapidly progressive renal failure. She had had 3 PEs without any complications. At the beginning of the 4th, she vomitted and had a c. v. collapse. An ECG was recorded which showed a third degree arterio-ventricular block. She had a cardiac arrest and could not be resuscitated.

There was no necropsy.

Case 6

A 70-year-old woman with mitral insufficiency had, after 31 of plasma had been exchanged, a fatal pulmonary edema.

No necropsy was performed, but a breaking of a mitral cord was presumed to be responsible for her death.

Case 7

A man with myasthenia gravis had a cardio pulmonary failure of which he died. A massive pulmonary embolism was found during necropsy.

Serious accidents complicated 0.5% of the PEs and occurred in 3.1% of the patients. One patient out of 147 died during or immediately after PE (0.7%).

Discussion

In order to obtain the greatest number of answers, we purposely wrote the questionnaires in the simplest way. They are, therefore, incomplete and some points are not considered, such as the relationship between replacement solution or clinical indication and side effects. We will reexamine this point later based on our own experience.

Frequency of Side Effects

There is no correlation between the number of PEs performed by each team (which could be considered as a reflection of its experience) and the frequency of side effects (which greatly differs from one team to another: 0–46%). This variation probably results from several factors (fig. 2):
(1) The experience of each team could not be simply reduced to the number of PEs performed.
(2) The systematic premedication used by some centers will certainly reduce the incidence of side effects, as will the preventive injections with calcium salts which are frequently performed.
(3) Specific recruitment of patients by each institute. However, with the exception of 2 centers, each team was concerned with a variety of indications. These 2 treat a single disease: solid tumors for one; hyperimmunized pregnant women for the other.
(4) The replacement solution used. 5 teams used a single relacement fluid

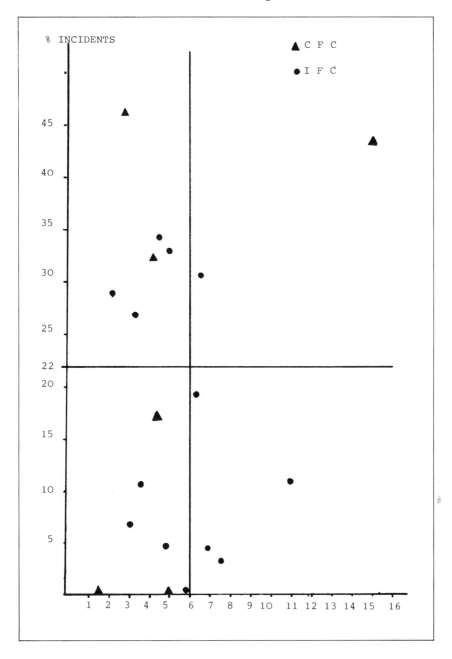

Fig. 2. Incidence of side effects according to the number of PE/patient, 1979.

(4 times FFP; 1 time serum human albumin). The other 14 teams used several solutions, generally in combination (FFP, lyophilised plasma, cryoprecipitate-depleted plasma, modified fluid gelatin, serum human albumin, crystalloids).

(5) The volume of plasma exchanged in each patient. This criteria was not included in our questionnaire.

(6) The number of PEs per patient. There seems to be no correlation between this parameter and the frequency of side effects (fig. 2).

(7) The way various clinical manifestations are recorded during PEs. This is certainly a point which varies from one team to another. An attempt at standardization could be made on the basis of a common surveillance document which everyone could use who performs PE.

(8) The type of cell separator used. None of the points we saw seemed to

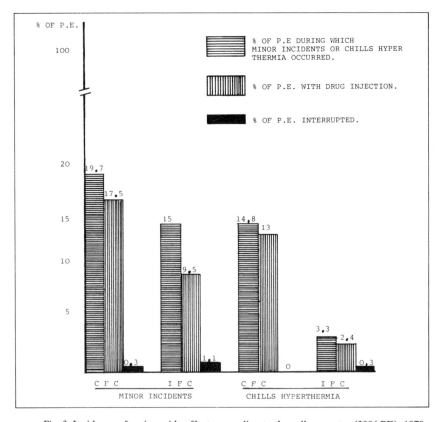

Fig. 3. Incidence of various side effects according to the cell separator (3086 PE), 1979.

be specific for any system: intermittent-flow centrifugation (IFC) or continuous-flow centrifugation (CFC). Minor side effects occur more frequently during continuous-flow centrifugation procedures (fig. 3). Unfortunately, the data collected cannot be submitted for statistical analysis, because the comparibility of the populations was not established (i. e. number of PE, frequency, volume, solutions, diagnosis, etc).

The questionnaire we sent was not detailed enough to allow us to appreciate the influence of the replacement solution, or the nature of the disease treated, on the clinical tolerance of PE. We will, therefore, briefly report our own experience on these 2 points, based on 400 PEs in 85 patients (all with intermittent-flow centrifugation).

(a) The Replacement Solution
We compared the tolerance of various replacement solutions of 2 groups in which patients were treated according to similar procedures with regard to frequency, volume, and number of PEs (tables IX and X). The only significant difference was between FFP and the combination of FFP and continuous-flow centrifugation in the cancerous group; and between FFP and the combination of FFP and serum human albumin in the noncancerous group.

Table IX. Frequencies of side effects according to the replacement solution. Patients with solid tumors

	FFP	MFG + FFP	MFG	HSA + FFP
No. of PE	171	88	7	8
Side effects (except serious accidents)	48 (28%)	34 (38.6%)	4 (57.1%)	5 (62.5%)

Table X. Frequencies of side effects according to the replacement solution. Non cancerous patients

	FFP	MFG + FFP	MFG	HSA + FFP
No. of PE	58	45	19	4
Side effects (except serious accidents)	10 (17.2%)	18 (40%)	5 (26.3%)	2 (50%)

(b) The Nature of the Disease Treated
We compared 171 PEs performed in cancerous patients (8) with 58 PEs in noncancerous patients (who had mainly connective tissue diseases). All exchanges were with FFP.
There were no significant difference in the frequency of side effects between these 2 groups.

Conclusion

It is obvious that the results presented here cannot be submitted to any statistical analysis because of their heterogeneity. The comparison of clinical results from different groups – the effect of the technical parameters (number, volume, frequency of PE) upon the efficiency of the exchange, or the influence of the plasma substitute upon the occurrence of side effects – will only become possible if comparative studies are performed, in which patients are selected on the same criteria and treated under the same technical conditions.

The frequency of accidents appearing here (considerably higher than usually thought) and the occurrence of death during or immediately after the exchange, are at variance with the general opinion that plasma exchange is a harmless procedure.

These facts must be considered before prescribing a PE treatment.

References

1 Baudelot, J.; Aufeuvre, J. P.; Cohen-Solal, M.; Esteves, A.: Technical aspects of repeated plasmapheresis and plasma exchanges and some of their clinical and biological consequences. In: Rosenfield; Serrou (eds.), Immune complexes and cancer patients, pp. 169–195 (Elsevier, North Holland 1981).
2 Bayer, W. L.; Farrales, F. B.; Summers, T.; Belcher, C.: Coagulation studies after plasma exchange with plasma protein fraction and lactated Ringer's solution. In: Goldman; Lowenthal (eds.), Leukocytes: Separation, collection, and transfusion, pp. 551–560 (Academic Press, London 1975).
3 Bussard, C. M.: The effects of intensive plasmapheresis on plasma constituents in donor and patients; PhD diss. Universität Bern (1979).
4 Bussel, A.: Etudes des incidents et accidents observés au cours de 250 échanges plasmatiques. Les Echanges Plasmatiques: Pratique, Résultats et Perspectives. (Bois Guillaume, March 1979).
5 Brossart, Y.: Incidents et accidents observés après 200 échanges plasmatiques chez 12 femmes enceintes, sévèrement RH immunisées. Les Echanges Plasmatiques: Pratique, Résultats et Perspectives. (Bois Guillaume, March 1979).

6 Flaum, M.; Cuneo, R. A.; Appelbaum, F. R.; Deisseroth, A. B.; King-Engel, W.; Gralnick, H. R.: The hemostatic imbalance of plasma-exchange transfusion. Blood. *54:* 694–702 (1979).

7 Gilcher, R. O.; Hashiba, U.: Automated plasmapheresis (coagulation studies). Haemonetics Proceedings of the Advanced Component Seminar, Boston 1977.

8 Israel, L.; Edelstein, R.; Mannoni, P.; Radot, E.; Greenspan, E. M.: Plasmapheresis in patients with disseminated cancer: Clinical results and correlation with changes in serum protein – The concept of 'non-specific blocking factors'. Cancer *40:* 3146–3154 (1977).

9 Keller, A. J.; Urbaniak, S. J.: Intensive plasma exchange on the cell separator: Effects on serum immunoglobulins and complement components. Br. J. Haemat. *38:* 531–540 (1978).

10 Keller, A. J.; Chirnside, A.; Urbaniak, S. J.: Coagulation abnormalities produced by plasma exchange on the cell separator with special reference to fibrinogen and platelet levels. Br. J. Haemat. *42:* 593–603 (1979).

11 Ocamica, P.: Applications thérapeutiques de la plasmaphérèse. Intérêt des échanges plasmatiques réalisés à l'aide de séparateurs de cellules sanguines dans l'épuration des protéines pathologiques. Thèse pour le Doctorat en médecine. Bordeaux (1979).

Dr. J. P. Aufeuvre, Centre Departemental de Transfusion Sanguine des Yvelines-Nord, 9, rue due Champ Gaillard, F-78302 Poissy-Cédex

II. General Tumor Immunology

Chairmen:
O. Goetze and *U. Kaboth*, Göttingen

Immune Mechanisms in Cancer

R. W. Baldwin

Cancer Research Campaign Laboratories,
University of Nottingham, Nottingham, Great Britain

Introduction

Immune responses elicited against tumor cells are highly complex and may involve the induction of specifically sensitized T-lymphocytes and/or antibody formation following recognition of tumor-associated antigens [1, 2, 38]. In addition to these putative specific recognition mechanisms, there is another host component involving activated macrophages and natural-killer cells which forms a 'natural resistance' to tumor cells [1, 24, 25]. Tumor-host interactions may also lead to the generation of suppressor lymphocytes and macrophages, and the development of humoral factors which may interfere with both specific and non-specific cellular interactions involved in anti-tumor mechanisms [6, 8, 35]. This includes the release of tumor antigen and/or immune complexes into the circulation and tumor cells, either directly, or indirectly through interactions with host cells, release immunosuppressive products [6].

Considering the therapeutic implications, there are several approaches where specific and/or non-specific intervention may be developed. This includes immunization with tumor antigen-containing vaccines so that the immunological manipulation leads to the enhancement of rejection mechanisms rather than suppression [1]. Alternately immunomodulating agents may be used to stimulate and/or activate natural immunity and these may also enhance specific immunity. A third approach to therapy might involve the removal or reduction of the array of factors, specific and non-specific, which interfere with host responses [35].

Immunological Recognition of Malignant Cells

The original evidence cited in identifying human tumor-associated antigens showed that peripheral blood lymphocytes from patients were cytotoxic *in vitro* when tested on cultured tumor cells, the reactivities indicating that many tumors exhibited tumor-type specific antigens [3]. These findings are now viewed as equivocal, since it has been shown that the microcytotoxicity test, which involves prolonged co-cultivation of tumor cells and lymphocytes, does not necessarily measure tumor-related reactivities [26]. Also there are now numerous studies showing that lymphocytes from normal healthy donors are cytotoxic for cultured tumor cells, this effect being mediated by natural-killer cells. Alternative approaches for identifying cell-mediated immunity to tumor-associated antigens have since been introduced. These include *in vivo* testing of the delayed hypersensitivity reaction induced in patients following cutaneous injection of tumor cells or extracts [44]. Several *in vitro* tests have also been developed, the leukocyte-migration inhibition and leukocyte-adherence inhibition assays having achieved some popularity. The leukocyte-adherence inhibition test measures the reduction of adherence of peripheral blood leukocytes from patients after exposure to tumor extracts and has been developed as a hemocytometer [22] or tube test [40]. Although these tests are relatively simple and easy to perform, there has been considerable variation in their successful application in studying cell-mediated immunity to human tumors. They also suffer from a lack of understanding of the immunological basis for the reduction in leukocyte adherence following antigen exposure.

Because of the general lack of acceptance of tests for cell-mediated immunity, there is a resurgence of interest in typing human-tumor antigens using antibody-binding assays. This approach has been particularly strengthened following the development of techniques for producing monoclonal antibodies to cell-surface antigens [32] and this clearly may render obsolete the use of antisera produced against tumor cells or extracts in xenogeneic hosts. In this technique, spleen cells from appropriately immunized mice are fused, using polyethylene glycol, with cells of a murine myeloma line. Following selection of hybridomas, those producing antibody are evaluated by testing culture supernatants and positive hybridomas cloned. In most cases, hybridomas are being produced by fusion of spleen cells from mice immunized with human tumor cells or extracts so that antibodies, detecting normal cell-surface antigens as well as tumor-associated antigens, will be produced. Accordingly, selection of hybridomas secreting antibody to tumor-associated antigens has to be made from the analysis of antibody reacting with a range of target cells. This approach is illustrated by studies on the reactivity of antibodies produced by two hybridomas following fusion of spleen cells from mice immunized against human osteogenic sarcoma cells derived from a cultured cell line. These hybridoma-produced monoclonal antibodies reacted with cells of the tumor used for immunization and also cells from three allogeneic osteogenic sarcomas. In comparison, the antibodies did not react with skin fibroblasts derived from the tumor donor and a range of other target cells. Notably, also, three other osteogenic sarcoma-derived target cells did not bind antibody. From this it can be concluded that the antibody preparations react with antigens associated with some, but not all, osteogenic sarcoma-derived cell lines with little or no cross-reactivity with other normal or tumor cells [16].

Several investigators have reported the production of monoclonal antibodies to melanoma-associated antigens by hybridomas derived from fusion of mouse myeloma cells and spleen cells from mice immunized with cultured melanoma cells or membrane fractions [10, 33, 45]. When one compares the reactivities of monoclonal antibodies produced by several investigators using mouse spleen cells, it is evident that a whole range of epitopes displaying different specificities and cross reactivities can be delineated. This includes melanoma-associated antigens showing complete or partial restriction to the cells used for immunization as well as common melanoma products. These antigenic specificities may not be expressed upon other tumors or normal cells. In addition, common tumor-associated antigens have been identified, these being expressed upon melanoma cells and other tumors whilst other antigens may be expressed upon both normal and malignant cells. Here it should be noted that several types of melanoma-associated antigen, have been identified by serological studies with melanoma patients' sera [39]. These include epitopes restricted to a single melanoma as well as antigens expressed upon a range of target cells derived from melanomas and other tumors. Further delineation of the myriad of products specified on melanoma cells, particularly by interaction with monoclonal antibody, is now to be expected.

Monoclonal antibodies specifying cell-surface antigens have been produced against other human tumors including carcinomas of colon [27], neuroblastoma [31] and leukemic cells [37]. Colon carcinoma-associated antigens have been specified by reaction with monoclonal antibodies produced against cells derived from colorectal carcinoma cell lines. The tumor antigens detected by these antibodies were identified upon a range of colon-carcinoma cells as well as cells derived from surgical specimens. Since these antibodies did not react at detectable levels with cells of other tumors or normal colonic mucosa cells, the evidence to date implies that the reagents specify a common colorectal cancer-associated antigen.

Effector Cells Involved in Tumor Recognition

A role for specifically sensitized T-lymphocytes in tumor rejection was originally deduced from transplantation studies with animal tumors which showed that tumor immunity could not be induced following immunization of T-cell-deprived animals, e. g. following thymectomy, whole-body irradiation, and reconstitution with bone-marrow cells depleted of T-cells. Also tumor-cell immunization of congenitally athymic (nude) animals in which T-cells are absent, or present in small numbers, does not lead to the development of tumor-specific immunity [4].

Adoptive transfer experiments have also been used to demonstrate a requirement for specifically sensitized T-lymphocytes in tumor rejection. For example, inhibition of tumor growth in 'Winn-type' assays where murine tumor cells are injected admixed with sensitized lymphocytes into normal compatible recipients, is abrogated by treatment of lymphocytes with antisera directed against mouse T-cell alloantigens (anti-Ly sera) and complement.

The identification of specific T-cell-mediated killing of human tumor cells has been hampered by a number of technical problems; particularly those associated with the preparation of suitable target tumor cells and effector cell purifications. This is illustrated by recent studies reportedly identifying T-cell-mediated killing of autologous lung tumor cells [42]. Rather than using cultured tumor cells as target cells, these were derived from surgical specimens and processed so as to remove contaminating host cells. With this refinement in technology, it was possible to detect cell-mediated cytotoxic reactions when peripheral blood lymphocytes were tested in a 4-h ^{51}Cr-release assay against autologous tumor cells whereas cells derived from normal lung tissue were resistant. The effector cells could not be defined unequivocally as T-lymphocytes since, although they were identified in E-rosette-forming populations, cells mediating antibody-dependent cytotoxicity and NK activity may be present. This approach has also been used to detect cell-mediated immunity to autologous melanoma cells except that established cell lines, rather than cells derived from disaggregated fresh tissue, were used and the cytotoxicity test measured the survival of (^{3}H) proline-labelled cells after exposure to lymphocytes for 40 h [34]. Again, whilst cell-mediated reactivity was demonstrated in 18 of 32 patients using autologous lymphocyte-tumor cell combinations, the effector cells could not be unequivocally identified as T-lymphocytes. These two examples emphasize the current dilemma in determining whether or not human tumors do elicit specific T-cell responses. It may next be feasible however to identify these effector-cell populations using monoclonal antibodies to human T-cell markers and these can then be separated using cell-sorting techniques.

Suppressor T-Cells

One of the most significant aspects of T-lymphocyte recognition of tumor-associated antigens, as with many other antigens, is the discovery that T-suppressor cells (Ts), rather than T-cells mediating tumor rejection (TK), may be induced [8, 35]. An extreme example of the powerful influence of Ts cells is provided by investigations on UV-induced murine tumors [17]. These tumors will not grow on transplantation to normal compatible mice, whereas irradiated mice reconstituted with lymphoid cells from UV-treated donors (as a source of Ts cells) accept syngeneic tumor grafts. Similarly, studies with the highly immunogenic murine Meth-A fibrosarcoma have demonstrated that T-cell-mediated immunosuppression is an important factor governing tumor growth [7].

Two distinct types of Ts cells have been identified in tumor-bearing animals [35]. One type suppresses specific tumor-immune responses generated against tumor-associated antigens. This is typified by the suppressor T-cell generated in mice bearing MCA-induced sarcomas which inhibit the expression of tumor immunity to the individually distinct neoantigens on these tumors [21]. In this case adoptive transfer of tumor-bearer spleen or thymus cells to mice immunized to the same sarcoma abrogate their capacity to reject tumor challenge whereas spleen cells from mice bearing an immunologically different sarcoma were ineffective. In this case there is conclusive evidence that soluble factors containing factors encoded by the I-J subregion of the murine Major Histocompatibility Complex (MHC) are involved in the suppression response [36].

Other suppressor T-cells in tumor-bearing animals have been identified which act non-specifically, so inhibiting a number of immune functions [35]. This includes impairment of the capacity of tumor-bearing mice to produce delayed hypersensitivity responses to chemical hypersensitizers such as 2,4-dinitrofluorobenzene [15]. Non-specific Ts cells have been detected also by their capacity to inhibit lymphocyte responses to antigens or mitogens [35]. This is illustrated by the suppression of the plaque-forming capacity of normal murine spleen cells following sensitization with sheep RBCs by Ts spleen cells derived from tumor-bearing mice [35]. Similarly, spleen cells from mice bearing the Lewis-lung carcinoma have been shown to suppress Con-A induced lymphocyte stimulation [12]. The pathways leading to this type of immunosuppression are still ill-defined although a role for soluble factors including prostaglandins has been proposed [14].

Suppressor T-lymphocytes have been identified in cancer patients, but in view of the difficulties in detecting tumor-specific responses, these cells have been widely assayed against a range of non-specific immune responses. For example, regional tumor-draining lymph-node cells from patients with urological tumors have been shown to contain suppressor-cell precursors which could be activated by Conconavalin A (Con A) which then inhibit the proliferative response of autologous lymphocytes to Con A [11]. Lymph-node cells derived from nodes draining colon carcinoma have also been found to suppress the response of autologous peripheral blood lymphocytes to stimulation with either Con A or PHA [42].

Akin with these studies identifying suppressor lymph-node lymphocytes, numerous investigations have also detected suppressor-cell activity in peripheral blood. This is exemplified by experiments demonstrating lymphocytes in peripheral blood of patients with various malignancies which exhibit suppressor-cell activity as assessed by their influence on the blastogenesis response of lymphocytes to PHA and Con A [28].

Suppressor cells have also been identified within tumor-infiltrating lymphocytes, again usually by assaying their capacity to inhibit the blastogenic response of autologous or allogeneic lymphocytes following mitogen stimulation. This approach is illustrated by experiments showing that lymphocytes separated from enzyme-disaggregated tumor samples obtained from patients with lung or breast carcinoma (TIL) suppressed the stimulation response of peripheral blood lymphocytes and this revealed a suppressor-cell population in all but one case with the tumor-derived lymphocytes. In addition there was evidence that TIL also inhibited the stimulation of blood lymphocytes by autologous tumor cells implicating tumor-directed inhibitory effects [43].

Suppressor Factors

The generation of antigen-specific T-cells with suppressor properties is generally recognized as a normal component in the regulation of the immune response following specific antigenic stimulation, so forming a series of regulatory circuits [9]. These effects may be mediated by soluble factors as already discussed in studies showing that T-cell factors can abrogate the specific immune response to tumor-associated antigens on murine sarcomas [21, 36]. In addition, tumor-specific antibody and/or circulating immune complexes containing tumor antigen may modulate a tumor-immune response. Regulation of the immune response by antibody is a highly complex process, one proposal being that the effects are controlled via a dynamic equilibrium between circulating antibody, antigen, and antigen-antibody complexes [41]. In this connection there is considerable evidence indicating that immune complexes are present in the serum from patients with a wide range of malignant tumors including melanoma, osteogenic sarcoma, carcinoma of the lung, breast, and colon, Hodgkin's disease, and leukemia [5, 6]. Circulating immune complexes have been detected using non-specific tests such as C_{1q} or conglutinin binding, complement consumption tests, and fixation to Raji or murine leukemia L1210 cells. At this time, there is no conclusive evidence that the immune complexes determined in these tests contain tumor-related products but a reduction in serum levels has been demonstrated in a number of investigations following tumor removal. Also it has been reported that the detection of serum-immune complexes in patients with malignant diseases correlates with a less favorable prognosis [5]. At this time it is premature to suggest that these serum-borne immune complexes in cancer patients can, or do, modulate anti-tumor responses. There is evidence, however, that immune complexes containing tumor-associated antigens are present in the serum of tumor-bearing animals which may influence cellular and humoral immunity to these determinants [5].

Finally the developing tumor may shed (secrete) a variety of soluble products which can interfere specifically or non-specifically with tumor immunity. This is typified by the identification of substances in ascitic

fluids from ovarian-cancer patients which non-specifically inhibit lymphocyte function as determined by their influence on mitogen-induced blastogenesis [29]. This factor was isolated in protein fractions containing
albumin and α-globulins and so may be related to the broad group of
immunosuppressive proteins including also α-fetoprotein, pregnancy-
associated α2-macroglobulins, and C-reactive protein [13, 20].

Conclusions

The role of specific and/or non-specific host-defense mechanisms in
immunity to tumors, particularly in the tumor-bearing host, are still poorly
understood [1, 2]. 'Non-specific' effector cells, especially natural-killer
cells [24, 25] are currently receiving considerable attention and some
would even question whether immune responses generated against tumor-
associated antigens play any role in resistance to human cancer. This
reaction has grown following studies indicating that many naturally arising
animal tumors do not elicit immune-rejection responses [30]. Added to
this is the fundamental observation that tumor incidences in immunologically deprived (T-cell deficient) animals are not different from those in
immunocompetent hosts. Against these arguments one is impressed with
the powerful influence of specific tumor immunity against a wide range of
animal tumors induced with extrinsic agents, especially when the induction of suppressor cells is impaired [7]. Furthermore, there are many
reports demonstrating cell-mediated and humoral-immune responses to
human tumors, such as for example, in malignant melanoma [39]. Clearly,
it is imperative to definitively characterize these putative human-tumor
antigens. The development of monoclonal antibodies for specifying
human tumor-associated antigens may go some way to this, since it will
then be possible to exchange reagents between laboratories.

The role of immunosuppressive factors in the tumor-bearing host on
the growth and metastatic spread of tumors also has to be taken into
account in both immunological and non-immunological methods of cancer
treatment. There are a number of pathways involved in the induction of
specific and non-specific suppressor lymphocytes and macrophages which
are activated by tumor [1, 2]. Added to this the developing tumor itself
may secrete tumor-related immunosuppressive substances or even lead to
the synthesis of host products which exhibit this property. The overall
response to these many factors may be a diminution of immune compe-

tence in cancer patients. This has led to the development of procedures which attempt to restore cellular immune functions. This includes treatment with thymosins and many other immunomodulating agents now including interferon [1, 19]. Conversely, manipulation of the levels of tissue localized or circulating immunosuppressive factors may influence host resistance to tumors. This has clearly been shown with respect to the influence of selective elimination of suppressor cells by cyclophosphamide on the induction of tumor immunity [18]. Apart from early studies on the influence of serum blocking/unblocking factors on growth of murine tumors [23], the influence of humoral immunosuppressive factors has not been explored in any detail and this surely needs to be developed with respect to clinical trials on plasmaphoresis.

Acknowledgments

These studies were supported by a grant from the Cancer Research Campaign, England.

References

1   Baldwin, R. W.: Immunotherapy of tumors. Cancer Chemother. Annu. *2:* 150–175 (1980).
2   Baldwin, R. W.: Mechanisms of immunity in cancer. Pathobiol. Annu. (in press, 1981).
3   Baldwin, R. W.; Embleton, M. J.: Assessment of cell mediated immunity to human tumor-associated antigens. Int. Rev. exp. Path. *17:* 49 (1977).
4   Baldwin, R. W.; Pimm, M. V.: Human tumour xenografts in athymic nude mice: Nonspecific host rejection responses. In: Sparrow (ed.), Immunodeficient Animals for Cancer Research, pp. 125–133 (Macmillan, London 1980).
5   Baldwin, R. W.; Robins, R. A.: Circulating immune complexes in cancer. In: Sell (ed.), Cancer Markers, pp. 507–531 (Humana Press, Clifton, N. J. 1980).
6   Baldwin, R. W.; Byers, V. S.; Robins, R. A.: Circulating immune complexes in cancer: Characterization and potential as tumour markers. Behring Inst. Mitt. *64:* 63 (1979).
7   Berendt, M. J.; North, R. J.: T-cell mediated suppression of anti-tumor immunity. An explanation for progressive growth of an immunogenic tumor. J. exp. Med. *151:* 69 (1980).
8   Broder, S.; Muul, L.; Waldmann, T. A.: Suppressor cells in neoplastic disease. J. natn. Cancer Inst. *61:* 5 (1978).
9   Cantor, H.: Control of the immune system by inhibitor and inducer T lymphocytes. Annu. Rev. Med. *30:* 269 (1979).
10   Carrel, S.; Accolla, R. S.; Carmagnola, A. L.; Mach, J.-P.: Common human melanoma-associated antigens detected by monoclonal antibodies. Cancer Res. *40:* 2523 (1980).
11   Catalona, W. J.; Ratiff, T. L.; McCool, R. E.: Concanavalin A-inducible suppressor cells in regional lymph nodes of cancer patients. Cancer Res. *39:* 4372 (1979).
12   Clerici, E.; Schechter, B.; Feldman, M.: Enrichment of suppressor cell activity by

hydrocortisone: Suppression of *in vitro* activation of splenocytes from mice bearing Lewis lung carcinoma. Int. J. Cancer *25:* 349 (1980).

13   Cooper, E. H.; Stone, J.: Acute phase reactant proteins in cancer. Adv. Cancer Res. *30:* 1 (1979).

14   Droller, M. J.; Lindgren, J. A.; Claessen, H.-E.; Perlmann, P.: Production of prosto-glandin E by bladder tumor cells in tissue culture and a possible mechanism of lympho-cyte inhibition. Cell Immunol. *47:* 261 (1979).

15   Elgert, K. D.: In vivo assessment of tumor-induced non-specific suppression of contact sensitivity. Cell. Immunol. *49:* 395 (1980).

16   Embleton, M. J.; Gunn, B.; Byers, V. S.; Baldwin, R. W.: Antigens on naturally arising animal and human tumors detected by monoclonal antibodies. Transplant. Proc. (in press, 1981).

17   Fisher, M. S.; Kripke, M.: Further studies on the tumor-specific suppressor cells induced by ultra violet radiation. J. Immunol. *121:* 1139 (1978).

18   Glaser, M.: Augmentation of specific immune response against a syngeneic SV40-induced sarcoma in mice by depletion of suppressor T cells with cyclophosphamide. Cell Immunol. *48:* 339 (1979).

19   Goldstein, A. L.; Low, T. L. K.; Thurman, G. B.; Zatz, M. M.; Hall, N.; Chen, C.-P.; Hu, S.-K.; Naylor, P. B.; McClure, J. E.: Current status of thymosin and other hor-mones of the thymus gland. Recent Prog. Horm. Res. (in press, 1981).

20   Goren, G.; Nelken, D.: Normal immunosuppressive proteins. Isolation of a glycopro-tein active fraction. Immunology *39:* 305 (1980).

21   Greene, M. I.; Perry, L. L.: Regulation of the immune response to tumor antigen. VI. Differential specificities of suppressor T cells or their products and effector T cells. J. Immunol. *121:* 2363 (1978).

22   Halliday, W. J.: Historical background and aspects of the mechanism of leukocyte adherence inhibition. Cancer Res. *39:* 558 (1979).

23   Hellström, K. E.; Hellström, I.; Nepom, J. T.: Serum blocking factors – are they important? B. B. A. Reviews on Cancer *473:* 121 (1978).

24   Herberman, R. B.: Natural cell mediated immunity against tumors, pp. 1–1360 (Academic Press, New York 1980).

25   Herberman, R. B.; Holden, H. T.: Natural cell mediated immunity. Adv. Cancer Res. *27:* 305 (1978).

26   Herberman, R. B.; Oldham, R. K.: Problems associated with study of cell-mediated immunity to human tumors by microcytotoxicity assays. J. natn. Cancer Inst. *55:* 749 (1975).

27   Herlyn, M.; Steplewski, Z.; Herlyn, D.; Koprowski, H.: Colorectal carcinoma-specific antigen: Detection by means of monoclonal antibodies. Proc. natn. Acad. Sci. USA *76:* 1438 (1979).

28   Hersh, E. M.; Patt, Y. Z.; Murphy, S. G.; Dirke, K.; Zander, A.; Adegbite, M.; Goldman, R.: Radiosensitive thymic hormone-sensitive peripheral blood suppressor cell activity in cancer patients. Cancer Res. *40:* 3134 (1980).

29   Hess, A. D.; Gall, S. A.; Dawson, J. R.: Partial purification and characterization of a lymphocyte inhibitory factor(s) in ascitic fluids from ovarian cancer patients. Cancer Res. *40:* 1842 (1980).

30   Hewitt, H. B.: The choice of animal tumors for experimental studies of cancer therapy. Adv. Cancer Res. *27:* 149 (1979).

31   Kennett, R. H.; Gilbert, F.: Myeloma producing antibodies against a human neuroblas-toma antigen present on fetal brain. Science. *203:* 1120 (1979).

32   Kennett, R. H.; Kearn, T. J. M.; Bechtal, K.: Monoclonal antibodies: A new dimension in biological analyses, pp. 1–422 (Plenum Press, New York 1980).

33   Koprowski, H.; Steplewski, Z.; Herlyn, D.; Herlyn, M.: Study of antibodies against human melanoma produced by somatic cell hybrids. Proc. natn. Acad. Sci. USA 75: 3405 (1978).
34   Livingston, P. O.; Shiku, H.; Bean, M. A.; Pinsky, C. M.; Oettgen, H. F.; Old, L. J.: Cell mediated cytotoxicity for cultured autologous melanoma cells. Int. J. Cancer 24: 34 (1979).
35   Naor, D.: Suppressor cells: Permitters or promoters of malignancy. Adv. Cancer Res. 29: 45–125 (1979).
36   Perry, L. L.; Benacerraf, B.; Greene, M. I.: Regulation of the immune response to tumor antigen. IV. Tumor antigen-specific suppressor factor(s) bear I-J determinants and induce suppressor T cells in vivo. J. Immunol. 121: 2144 (1978).
37   Ritz, J.; Pesando, J. M.; Notis-McConarty, J.; Lazarus, H.; Schlossman, S. F.: A monoclonal antibody to human acute lymphoblastic leukaemia antigen. Nature 283: 583 (1980).
38   Rosenberg, S. A.: Serologic analysis of human cancer antigens, pp. 1–712 (Academic Press, New York 1980).
39   Shiku, H.; Takahashi, T.; Resnick, L. A.; Oettgen, H. F.; Old, L. J.: Cell surface antigens of human malignant melanoma, III. Recognition of autoantibodies with unusual characteristics. J. exp. Med. 145: 784 (1977).
40   Shuster, J.; Thomson, D. M. P.; Gold, P.: Immunodiagnosis. In: Castro (ed.), Immunological Aspects of Cancer, pp. 284–312 (M. T. P. Press, Lancaster, England 1978).
41   Theofilopoulas, A.: Immune complexes in humoral immune responses: Suppressive and enhancing effects. Immunology Today 1: 1 (1980).
42   Vose, B. M.: Specific T cell killing of autologous lung tumour cells. Cell. Immunol. 55: 12 (1980).
43   Vose, B. M.; Moore, M.: Heterogeneity of suppressors of mitogen responsiveness in human malignancy. Cancer Immunol. Immunother. 9: 163–171 (1980).
44   Weese, J. L.; Herberman, R. B.; Hollinshead, A. C.; Cannon, G. B.; Keels, M.; Kibrite, A.; Morales, A.; Char, D. H.; Oldham, R. K.: Specificity of delayed cutaneous hypersensitivity reactions to extracts of human tumor cells. J. natn. Cancer Inst. 60: 255 (1978).
45   Yeh, M.-Y.; Hellström, I.; Brown, J. P.; Warner, G. A.; Hansen, J. A.; Hellström, K. E.: Cell surface antigens of human melanoma identified by monoclonal antibody. Proc. natn. Acad. Sci. USA 76: 2927 (1979).

R. W. Baldwin, MD, Cancer Research Campaign Laboratories, University of Nottingham, GB-Nottingham NG7 2RD

Serum-Blocking Factors in Tumor Host. Are They Important?

S. C. Bansal and B. R. Bansal

New Delhi, India

Introduction

Tumor-host relationship is very complex. Yet knowledge acquired in the recent past permits one to draw certain conclusions, which are

(1) The tumor cells, though characterized by membrane alterations, may lack tumor-rejection antigens [25];

(2) Not all membrane alterations in the tumor cells may be recognized by the immune system of the host and the process of recognition may itself be dependent on the genetic constitution of the host [25];

(3) Both experimental tumors in animals and spontaneous tumors in humans exhibit a weak antigenic response in the host of origin [2, 5, 20];

(4) A failure in effector mechanism of the tumor host in rejecting tumor may be due to either a decline in the immunocompetence of the host with the establishment and growth of tumor [22] and/or appearance of serum factors capable of inhibiting antitumor cellular immunity (table I) [20, 21].

At present a great deal of interest is being shown in the possibility that host-immune mechanisms fail to effectively attack the tumor cells in vivo. Interest in such mechanisms was evoked by the fact that serum-blocking factors (SBF) were present in tumor bearer but not in tumor-free

Abbreviations
SBF – Serum-blocking factors
DMH – Dimethylhydrazine dihydrochloride
GI – Gastrointestinal
ATG – Antithymocyte globulin

Table I. Possible immunological mechanisms affecting tumor growth

Promotors	Inhibitors
humoral	
Suppressor molecules	Antitumor antibodies (IgM-Ab)
Antitumor antibodies (IgG-Ab)	(Ab + complement)
Aggregated IgG	(Ab + lymphocytes)
Free tumor antigens	
Antigen-antibody complexes (Ag-Ab)	
cellular	
Suppressor cells	Immune lymphocytes 'T'
('T' lymphocytes)	Immune macrophages
Blocking Ab producing cells	Non-immune lymphocytes
('B' lymphocytes)	(natural-killer cells)
	'B' lymphocytes
	(Ab-dependent)
	Tumor-host relationship

host [19], which partially explained the paradox of coexistance of anti-tumor cellular immunity and tumor growth [2, 5]. The importance of SBF was further strengthened by the discovery that administration of serum, capable of counteracting the serum-blocking activity in vitro, caused tumor rejection in several tumor models [11–13]. Inspite of the fact that it has been more than a decade since the existence of SBF in tumor bearers was described neither their exact nature nor the mechanism of production has been clearly defined [2, 5].

In this presentation we will discuss evidence for:

(1) Presence of antitumor immunity in vivo in an autochthonous tumor host;

(2) The importance of SBF in a tumor host;

(3) A clinically feasible ex vivo immunoabsorption procedure, which can lead to a decrease in SBF in a tumor host;

(4) That multimodal immune manipulation may be an optimal immunotherapeutic approach.

Evidence for the Presence of Antitumor Immunity in Vivo in an Autochthonous Host

Clinical experience indicates that a patient from whom a tumor has been successfully removed is at a higher risk of developing a successive primary tumor of the same organ and/or of other organs [14, 15]. Further, established tumors develop from subclinical metastatic foci after a prolonged disease-free interval [14]. Although a higher risk in paired organs may be argued on the basis that similar tissues were previousely exposed to the same carcinogenic factors [15], the development of subsequent tumors in the same organ, in face of antitumor immunity, makes one doubt the efficacy of immune system in an autochthonous host. Studies which can delineate the role of host-defense mechanisms and explain those observations will be of importance [3, 15].

Dimethylhydrazine (DMH)-induced colon carcinomas in rats have been claimed to resemble, both histologically and immunologically, colon neoplasms in humans [17]. We therefore selected this tumor model to examine the effectiveness of antitumor immunity in vivo, induced by the first primary tumor against nascent tumors in an autochthonous host. The method of tumor induction in rats using DMH and the diagnosis of gastrointestinal (GI) tumors by the direct visualization or laparotomy has been described in detail [10]. The experimental design and results are given in figure 1. Briefly, a group of 39 rats of similar age, weight, and sex were exposed to identical carcinogenic dosage of DMH and were randomly divided into four groups as follows:

Group A – The first tumor observed in each rat was left in situ;

Group B – The first tumor observed in each rat of this group was left in situ in an isolated segment with an intact blood supply;

Group C – The first tumor observed in each rat of this group was excised and an end to end anastmosis of the GI tract was performed;

Group D – The first tumor observed in each rat of this group was excised and an end to end anastomosis of the GI tract was performed. In addition all rats of group D received an immunorepressive dosage of antithymocyte globulin (ATG-rabbit antirat).

The rats of group A and B continued to develop multiple GI tumors. A total of 13 and 12 successive GI tumors were observed in rats of group A and B, whereas only 2 new primary GI tumors were detected in rats of group C (p < 0.05 as compared to either group A or B). However, 7 additional GI tumors were observed in 6 out of 10 rats in group D (p < 0.05 when compared to group C). All rats of group A and B died of widespread metastatic tumors, on the other hand, none of the rats in group C developed metastasis (p < 0.01). However immunosuppression with ATG (group D) facilitated the development of metastasis in 5 out of 10 rats (p < 0.05 when compared to group C). Furthermore the number

Groups (number of rats)	Status of first GI tumor	Number of GI tumors when first diagnosed	Number of additional GI tumors (observation period in days)	Number of rats with metastasis	Mucosal abnormalities (premalignant)
A (10)	Tumor ⟶ in situ 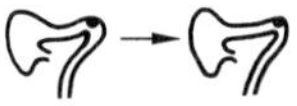	10	13 (280-380)	10	9
B (9)	Tumor ⟶ in isolated segment of colon 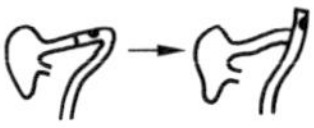	10	12 (340-380)	9	9
C (10)	Tumor ⟶ excised, end to end anastomosis 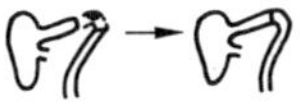	10	2* (380-480)	0*	3+
D (10)	Tumor ⟶ excised, end to end anastomosis + ATG 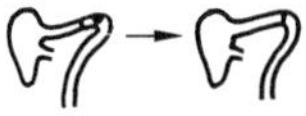	10	7 (380-400)	5	10

* p < 0.01 when compared to group A and B
+ p < 0.05 when compared to group A, B and D.

Fig. 1. Antitumor immunity in an autochthonous host: Experimental design and results.

of mucosal abnormalities capable of developing into invasive malignancies [10] was higher in rats of group A, B and D when compared to those of group C. Our results in this tumor model suggest that removal of a primary tumor can confer effective specific antitumor immunity in an autochthonous host. It is recognized that the primary immunizing tumor in each rat was in its early stage of development, since all tumor excised from rats of group C and D were less than 4 mm in size and had not invaded beyond lamina propria. Blood lymphocytes obtained prior to and after tumor excision from each rat of group C and D exhibited specific cytotoxic effect on colon carcinoma cells.

It is of importance to identify the reasons for the development of successive tumors in an autochthonous host in the face of demonstrable antitumor immunity. Several mechanisms to explain this breakdown of the restraints imposed by the host's immune system have been suggested which include (table I):

(1) Inhibition of cellular immunity by free antigens continuously being shed by the tumors [1] or by complexes formed by the antitumor antibodies and free antigens [27, 28];

(2) Development of suppressor cells in the presence of continuous stimuli by the tumor antigens [21];

(3) Production of factors by the growing tumors toxic to lymphoid tissue of the host;

(4) A breakdown in cellular immunity due to reasons unexplained, which, in our experiments, was iatrogenically produced by inoculation with ATG. Delineation of mechanisms may suggest the means to counteract them.

At present, for therapeutic purposes, it may be prudent to attack all such mechanisms simultaneously. It is of significance that 2 rats in group C and 5 rats in group D, which developed additional GI tumors, had persisting serum-blocking activity after the excision of the first tumor, whereas the serum obtained after excision of the first tumor from each of the remaining 8 rats in group C was free of blocking activity [3 and unpublished data].

Blocking and Unblocking Factors in Tumor Host

The possibility that an antibody in body fluids may be inimical to tumor host and may allow tumor growth was suspected by *Hodenpyl* in 1910 [23]. He further postulated the presence of factors capable of causing tumor destruction in the body fluids of patients with spontaneous tumor regression. He utilized these principles in treating patients with breast carcinomas. Unfortunately, a detailed description of these patients is not available. This might well be an early postulation of the concept of blocking and unblocking serum factors in tumor hosts.

Blocking of sensitized lymphocyte-mediated cytotoxic effects by serum from host with progressively growing Moloney sarcoma (progressor serum) but not from host with regressed tumors (regressor serum) was first shown in vitro using colony inhibition assay [19, 20]. Since then, the specificity and presence of blocking-serum activity has been shown to exist in many experimental animal-tumor systems as well as in humans with growing tumors [2, 5, 20]. Investigations to determine whether or not blocking serum factors play a significant role in a tumor host have led to the following conclusions:

(1) The appearance of blocking activity is an early rather than a late phenomenon in tumor development [12, 27];

(2) Blocking activity rapidly disappears upon complete tumor excision, whereas the continuous presence of blocking activity correlates with the development of subsequent palpable tumors from nascent tumors [10, 12, 27];

(3) When a second test-tumor graft is given to an animal soon after a total excision of a growing tumor, the blocking activity persists, even though the second graft is not yet palpable [27];

(4) It can be demonstrated that tumor eluate or sera from tumor hosts can enhance tumor growth in an immunologically intact host [9];

(5) Administration of serum capable of counteracting the serum-blocking activity (unblocking serum is an operational term) can cause tumor regression. However, the use of unblocking serum alone, for rejecting well-established tumors, has never been studied [11].

The nature of these blocking-serum factors has not been agreed upon. Under different test conditions it can be demonstrated that tumor antigen alone [1], specific antigen-antibody complexes [2, 28], and aggregated antitumor antibodies [26] can inhibit specific cellular immunity. Perhaps all three mechanisms are operational in vivo and their relative importance remains to be defined [2, 5].

A Clinically Feasible ex Vivo Immunoabsorption Procedure, which Can Lead to a Decrease in SBF in a Tumor Host

On the basis of observations mentioned above it has been repeatedly suggested that the role of SBF in a tumor host can best be evaluated from experiments designed to specifically remove these suppressive factors from the body fluids of tumor hosts. However, the experience with the use of specific or nonspecific immunoabsorbent in an extra-corporeal circulation is limited [5, 6]. Protein A, a molecule present on the wall of certain strains of S. aureus, has the biological property of interacting and binding the Fc portion of mammalian IgG [29] and its complexes [24]. Further, protein A molecule can absorb blocking activity from serum of a tumor host and render the absorbed serum cytotoxic to specific tumor cells [30]. We proposed a system consisting of a plasma separator and membrane filters in which intact S. aureus organisms, heat killed, and formalin stabilized, can be safely used to remove IgG from plasma of human beings in an extracorporeal circulation. This system was applied to 19 dogs who where subjected to a total of 58 procedures. Except for minor changes in the dogs' electrocardiograms and blood pressures, no significant alterations in functions of vital organs were recorded, thus establishing the safety of this procedure [6]. So far we have tested the immunotherapeutic effects of this procedure on 3 dogs bearing different types of tumors and 2 human patients with wide-spread metastasis from colon carcinoma. The detailed results describing the antitumor effects of this procedure on above-mentioned tumor hosts have been published previously [7, 8]. Briefly, the repeated removal of IgG and its complexes using S. aureus resulted in:

(1) Decrease in serum-blocking activity and immune complexes;
(2) Decrease in tumor mass;
(3) Histological evidence of tumor destruction;
(4) Potentiation of existing antitumor immunity.

Our experiences with dogs and humans clearly demonstrate the feasibility of using immunoabsorbents in ex vivo circulation for the treatment of not only patients with tumors but several types of clinical situations such as auto-immune diseases and removal of blood-group antibodies or performed antibodies in a transplantation recipient etc. However, we should point out that the procedure is technically complex and expensive to undertake on a large number of patients [8]. Fortunately, protein A can be bound to several substrates such as silica, sepharose (Pharmacia Fine Chemicals, Sweden), and plastics etc. which substitute the use of S. aureus therefore eliminating the need of filtration system [8]. Further work, using polymers of inert porous plastics as a substrate to attach protein A, is needed so that either the absorption can be performed on whole blood in an ex vivo circulation thus avoiding separation of plasma; or prefered yet the immunoabsorption could be carried out entirely in vivo. Preliminary experiences tend to support the latter procedure, although a detailed account is beyond the scope of this article.

Multimodal Immune Manipulation: An Optimal Approach to Immunotherapy

Among several immunological alterations in a host with growing tumor, 2 defects stand out in particular:

Table II. Multimodal therapy in DMH-induced GI tumors in rats: Experimental design and results

Groups (number of rats)	Therapy-dosage (intravenous) Splenectomy C. parvum (CP) Unblocking serum (US) Unblocked lymphocytes (UL) Levamisole (LMS)	Number of rats with GI tumors on day			Number of total GI tumors on day			Number of rats with metastasis on day			Histologic evidence of tumor rejection	
		180	300	390	180	300	390	180	300	390	Mild to mod.	Severe
A (10)	No treatment	3	10	10	4	20	21	0	6	10	18	0
B-1 (8)	Splenectomy											
B-2 (10)	Absorbed rabbit serum 1.0 ml./dose × 45	5	18	18	6	32	35	0	11	15	–	–
C (8)	Splenectomy CP-0.1 mg./dose × 9	2	8	8	2	12	19	0	2	8	17	0
D (8)	Splenectomy CP-0.1 mg./dose × 9 US-1.0 ml./dose × 45	3	8	8	3	10	12	0	0	1[+]	7	8[++]
E (10)	CP-0.1 mg./dose × 9 US-1.0 ml./dose × 45 UL-2.0 × 10^7 cells/dose × 9 LMS-1.0 mg./dose × 9	4	8	6*	5	9*	6*	0	0	0*	3	4[++]

(18 — indicated at group B-1/B-2)

[+] p < 0.05 or better, when compared with group A, B and C
* p < 0.05 or better, when compared to group A and C
[++] p < 0.05 or better, when compared to group A and B

(1) Decline in immunocompetence with the establishment and growth of malignant tumor [22] and

(2) Appearance of factors capable of modulating antitumor immune responses [5].

Based on these observations we suggested that combining the removal or counteraction of serum-blocking factors by bolstering specific or nonspecific antitumor immunity would yield optimal antitumor effects [4].

We studied the immunotherapeutic effects of multiple immune manipulation in a DMH-induced rat GI tumor model [4]. The multimodal immune manipulation consisted of:

(1) Unblocking serum, antitumor serum capable of counteracting serum-blocking activity;

(2) Unblocked lymphoid cells, extensively washed lymphocytes [15, 16];

(3) C. parvum, a stimulant of macrophages;

(4) Levamisole, an immunotropic agent.

The experimental conditions and results are described in table II. The rats in groups subjected to multimodal therapy as compared to those treated with one therapy only showed significant tumor inhibition, and did not develop regional and distant metastasis. Histological evidence of severe tumor destruction was present in all tumors of rats subjected to multimodal immunotherapy [4]. In as many as 5 out of 7 tumors from rats treated with multimodal manipulation, the tumorous areas of GI tract were covered with normal appearing mucosa, suggesting that the mucosa in these areas had reverted to normal [4]. With such results we strongly feel that ex vivo immunoabsorption with protein A combined with C. parvum and levamisole may yield superior therapeutic effects and merit experimental trials.

References

1   Alexander, P.: Escape from immune destruction by the host through shedding of surface antigens: Is this characteristic shared by malignant cell and embryonic cells? Cancer Res. 34: 2077 (1974).

2   Baldwin, R. W.; Robbins, R. A.: Humoral factors abrogating cell-mediated immunity in the tumor-bearing host. Curr. Top. Microbiol. Immunology 72: 21–53 (1975).

3   Bansal, B. R.; Mark, R.; Mobini, J.; Rhoads, J. E.; Bansal, S. C.: Demonstration of effective antitumor immunity in an autochthonous host bearing 1,2-dimethylhydrazine induced primary-colon tumors. J. natn. Cancer Inst. 63: 127–132 (1978).

4   Bansal, B. R.; Mobini, J.; Bansal, S. C.: Multimodal immunotherapy of primary gas-
     trointestinal tumors in rats. 1. Histologic correlation. Cancer 42: 2079–2096 (1978).
5   Bansal, S. C.; Bansal, B. R.; Boland, J. P.: Blocking and unblocking serum factors in
     neoplasia. Curr. Top. Microbiol. Immunology 72: 45–76 (1976).
6   Bansal, S. C.; Bansal, B. R.; Rhoads, J. E.; Cooper, D. R.; Boland, J. P.; Mark, R.: Ex
     vivo removal of mammalian immunoglobulin G; Method and immunologic alterations.
     Int. J. artif. Organs 1: 94–103 (1978).
7   Bansal, S. C.; Bansal, B. R.; Thomas, H. L.; Siegal, P. O.; Rhoads, J. E.; Cooper, D.
     R.; Terman, D. S.; Mark, R.: Ex vivo removal of serum IgG in a patient with colon
     carcinoma. Some biochemical, immunological, and histological observations. Cancer
     42: 1–18 (1978).
8   Bansal, S. C.; Bansal, B. R.; Husberg, B.; Lindstrom, C.; Nylander, G.; Mark, R.;
     Sjogren, H. O.: Use of biological immunoabsorbents in the treatment of tumor host.
     In: Therapeutic Plasma and Cytapheresis. Mono. Nat. Cancer Inst. (in print, 1981).
9   Bansal, S. C.; Hargreaves, R.; Sjogren, H. O.: Facilitation of polyoma tumor growth in
     rats by blocking sera and tumor eluate. Int. J. Cancer. 9: 97–108 (1972).
10   Bansal, S. C.; Mark, R.; Bansal, B. R.; Rhoads, J. E.: Immunologic surveillance against
     chemically induced primary colon carcinoma in rat. J. natn. Cancer Inst. 60: 667–675
     (1978).
11   Bansal, S. C.; Sjogren, H. O.: Counteraction of the blocking of cell-mediated tumor
     immunity by inoculation of unblocking sera and splenectomy: Immunotherapeutic
     effects on primary polyoma tumors in rats. Int. J. Cancer 9: 490–509 (1972 a).
12   Bansal, S. C.; Sjogren, H. O.: Correlation between changes in antitumor immune
     parameters and tumor growth in vivo in rats. Fed. Proc. 32: 165–172 (1972 b).
13   Bansal, S. C.; Sjogren, H. O.: Regression of polyoma tumor metastasis by combined
     unblocking and BCG treatment: Correlation with induced alterations in tumor immu-
     nity status. Int. J. Cancer 12: 179–193 (1973).
14   Berg, J. W.; Schottenfeld, D.; Ritter, F.: Incidence of multiple primary cancers. III
     cancers of the respiratory and upper digestive system as multiple primary cancers. J.
     natn. Cancer Inst. 44: 263–274 (1970).
15   Devitte, J. E.; Rothmoyo, L. A.; Brown, F. N.: The significance of multiple adenocar-
     cinoma of the colon and rectum. Ann. Surg. 169: 364–367 (1969).
16   Doyle, J. S.; Bell, J.; Deasy, P.; Thornes, R. D.: Activation or unblocking of T lympho-
     cytes. Lancet ii: 959–960 (1974).
17   Haase, P.; Cowen, D. M.; Knowles, J. C.; Cooper, E. H.: Evaluation of dimenthylhy-
     drazine-induced tumors in mice as a model system for colorectal cancer. Br. J. Cancer
     28: 530–543 (1973).
18   Hattler, B. G.; Soehnlein, B.: Inhibition of tumor-induced lymphocyte blastogenesis by
     a factor or factors associated with leucocytes. Science 184: 1374–1375 (1974).
19   Hellstrom, I.; Hellstrom, K. E.: Studies on cellular immunity and its serum-mediated
     inhibition in Moloney virus-induced mouse sarcomas. Int. J. Cancer 4: 587–600
     (1969).
20   Hellstrom, K. E.; Hellstrom, I.: Lymphocyte-mediated cytotoxicity and blocking serum
     activity to tumor antigens. Adv. Immunol. 18: 209–274 (1974).
21   Hellstrom, K. E.; Hellstrom, I.: Cell-mediated immunity to mouse tumors: Some
     recent findings. Ann. N. Y. Acad. Sci. 276: 165–175 (1976).
22   Hersh, E. M.; Gutterman, J. U.; Mavligit, G. M.; Mountain, C. W.; McBride, C. M.;
     Burgess, M. A.: Immunocompetence, immunodeficiency, and progress in cancer. Ann.
     N. Y. Acad. Sci. 276: 389–395 (1976).
23   Hodenpyl, E.: Treatment of carcinoma with body fluids of a recovered case. Med. Rec.
     359–360 (Feb. 1910).

24 Kessler, S. W.: Rapid isolation of antigens from cells with a staphylococcal protein A antibody absorbent: Parameters of the interaction of antibody-antigen complexes with protein A. J. Immun. *115:* 1617–1624 (1975).

25 Klein, G.: Immunological surveillance against neoplasia. The Harvey Lecture Series 69 (Academic Press, New York 1975).

26 Saksela, E.; Penttinen, K.; Pyrohonen, S.: Nonspecific blocking of human ovarian carcinoma-associated cellular cytotoxicity in vitro. Scand. J. Immunol. *3:* 781–788 (1974).

27 Sjogren, H. O.; Bansal, S. C.: Antigens in virally induced tumors. In: Amos (ed.), Progress in Immunology, pp. 921–938 (Academic Press, New York 1971).

28 Sjogren, H. O.; Hellstrom, I.; Bansal, S. C.; Hellstrom, K. E.: Suggestive evidence that 'blocking antibodies' of tumor-bearing individuals may be antigen-antibody complexes. Proc. natn. Acad. Sci. *68:* 1372–1375 (1971).

29 Sjoquist, J.: Structure and immunology of protein A. In: Jeljaszewics, Hryiewicks (eds.), 'Staphylococci and staphylococcal infection'. pp. 83–92 (S. Karger, Basel 1973).

30 Steel, G.; Ankerst, J.; Sjogren, H. O.: Alterations in in vitro antitumor activity of tumor-bearing serum by absorption with S. aureus. Cowan I. Int. J. Cancer *14:* 83–92 (1974).

S. C. Bansal, MD, D-131 Panchsheel Enclave, New Delhi, India

Immunotherapy of Cancer: Extracorporeal Adsorption of Plasma-Blocking Factors Using Nonviable Staphylococcus Aureus Cowan I

P. K. Ray, L. Clarke, D. McLaughlin, P. Allen, A. Idiculla, R. Mark, J. E. Rhoads, Jr., J. G. Bassett, D. R. Cooper

Departments of Surgery and Pathology, The Medical College of Pennsylvania and Hospital, Philadelphia, USA

Several reports [1–4] have indicated that antigenic tumors can grow *in vivo,* in spite of the presence of specifically sensitized lymphocytes in the host. These lymphocytes show antitumor cytotoxicity *in vitro,* but they cannot function internally because of the presence of immunosuppressive factors [5–11]. Lymphocyte effects are inhibited by suppressor cells [5, 6, 10, 11] and also by soluble plasma-blocking factors [5–9]. Certain specific plasma-blocking factors have been identified as an antigen [9], antibody [12–14], and antigen-antibody complex [8, 15], but some nonspecific plasma-blocking factors have also been identified [16].

Antigen-antibody complexes have been suspected of playing a role in the induction of tolerance for allografts [17] and in the maintenance of that tolerance [18]; also of being a contributing factor to immunosuppression in cancer [19]. The exact mechanism of immune complex-induced suppression of immune response is not fully understood. Several reports indicate that immune complexes may bind to the Fc-receptors on (a) target tumor cells, masking the antigenic sites [20]; (b) effector lymphocytes, preempting their reactivities against the tumor cells [20]; or (c) suppressor T-cells, activating their suppressor effects [6, 20–22]. Immune complexes have been suspected of having the ability to inhibit the killer-cell activity [20, 23, 24] and antibody-dependent cell-mediated cytotoxicity [24]. Thus, plasma immune complexes, in a tumor-bearing host, appear to have a predominant role in blocking the immune reactivities of the host, perhaps enabling tumors to adapt to the hostile immune environment of the host. It would be reasonable to expect, therefore, that abrogation of plasma-blocking factors (immune complexes and other blocking agents) would alter and/or inhibit the course of tumor growth through augmentation of the immune response of the host against the tumor.

Several methods for counteracting or removing the serum-blocking factors have been proposed [16, 25–34], and some have been tested experimentally in human beings to study their therapeutic implications [26, 28, 32–36].

Protein A of *Staphylococcus aureus* (SPA) Cowan I can bind the Fc-portion of immunoglobulin-G [37]. The binding of complexed IgG occurs more readily than binding of monomeric IgG by SPA, because of its capacity for multipoint attachment [38]. Binding of immune complexes (IC) with SPA is extremely rapid [39], whereas free IgG binding is comparatively slower [39]. It has been reported that SPA has greater affinity for serum IC than does free IgG [24].

Since 1978, we have been conducting investigations, exploiting this unique property of SPA, to adsorb myeloma IgG [40] and autoimmune antibodies [41, 42] from patients' plasma in an extracorporeal perfusion system. We have also been able to adsorb plasma-blocking factors, using SPA adsorbent from (1) 7,12 dimethyl-benz-anthracene-induced primary mammary adenocarcinomas in Sprague Dawley rats [27, 29, 31, 33]; (2) dogs bearing spontaneoulsly occurring tumors and transmissible venereal tumors [30, 33]; and (3) a large number of different types of cancer patients [32–34]. We have observed tumor regressions, following plasma adsorption over SPA, in the case of rat and dog tumors, and also in the case of human tumors. In this report we would like to review some of our experiences with respect to: (1) treating advanced human cancer patients; (2) hemodynamic changes during the immunoadsorption process; and (3) immunological and clinical response of patients to the treatment.

Materials and Methods

Patients

All of the patients we have treated so far have had a large tumor burden; all have had metastasized tumors, and all have received conventional treatments earlier. They were referred to us by physicians from many areas of the United States.

Patient Selection

All patients are evaluated immunologically and clinically. Patients who, in general, satisfy our selection criteria are included in the program. Those who are considered to be suitable for reasonably long-term follow up are given preference over others; however, we have treated some very sick patients in order to learn whether any benefit can be detected.

Staphylococcus Aureus Suspension

In our study, *Staphylococcus aureus* Cowan I has been used as the immunoadsorbent after subjecting it to heat and formalin treatment. The details of the preparation have been described elsewhere [41–42].

Collection of Plasma and Serum

From the patients studied, plasma and serum specimens were collected from heparinized or clotted whole blood by centrifuging at 1000 rpm for 30 min. The supernatant was separated and stored at $-20°$ C until tested. Plasma samples were drawn before and after the immunoadsorption procedure for various subsequent laboratory tests.

Evaluation of Immunoglobulins in the Plasma and Serum

Quantitative immunogel diffusion kits (Helena Laboratories, Beaumont, Texas) were used for estimating the concentration of human immunoglobulins and several other plasma proteins.

Immunoadsorption of Plasma in Cancer Patients

In order to draw blood, catheters were established in the femoral vein. The blood was returned through the vein in the arm. The heparinized blood was pumped through a cell separator and centrifuged as described earlier [28, 33, 34, 40–42]. The separated plasma was then pumped through a bacterial filter (0.2μ) containing *S. aureus* (0.5 g/kg body weight) suspension. The adsorbed plasma was reunited with the blood cells and returned through the vein of the patient. The details of the procedure have been described elsewhere [28, 33, 34, 40–42].

Results

Clinical Changes in Patients Receiving Immunoadsorption (IA) Treatment

The pattern of clinical changes observed in treatments was similar in almost all of the patients treated. During each IA procedure, the vital signs were monitored every 5–10 min during and after the procedure until they were stable. Oral temperature was taken every 30 min. During every run the patient showed varying degrees of hypovolemia 10–15 min after the initiation of the run. This was corrected by fluid replacement and/or intravenous transfusion of human serum albumin (12.5%). After 20–30 min, the systolic blood pressure rose gradually to about 160–180 mm of Hg. After about 45 min to 1 h, the patient started to shake. Some patients complained about some pain in the tumor area [34]. There was an increase in the temperature on the surface of the tumor by 1–2° C [34], followed by an increase in body temperature which varied in the range of 39–40° C. The procedure did not cause major discomfort to the patients, except for chills and shaking. A few patients experienced nausea. As of this writing, we have done over 200 IA procedures in human patients without occurrence of extreme morbidity. Elevated blood pressure and body temperature subsided to normal levels within 4–6 h. Usually there was no need for any drug to control these conditions.

Effect of Immunoadsorption Treatment in Metastatic Colon Carcinoma Patients

Case 1

A 55-year-old black female was presented with complaints of sharp pain in her umbilicus. She was treated by the IA procedure for a total of 15 treatments, over a period of 3 months. Our data indicated a decreased level of plasma immunoglobulin G (IgG), immune complexes (IC), and carcinoembryonic antigen (CEA) during the course of the treatment. Histopathological study of biopsied sections, taken during the course of the treatment, indicated tumor necrosis and fibrosis of tumor tissue, neovascularization, and lymphocyte infiltration. The patient experienced both subjective and objective positive clinical response, without extreme morbidity. The patient underwent surgery following the 15 IA treatments; she lived for 18 months post-treatment. 7 months after the IA treatment, she developed some problems and went to her oncologist for chemotherapy for a few months. After that she was unwilling to take therapy of any kind and died from metastatic carcinoma of the lung. The details of treatment of this patient and her response have been described elsewhere [34].

Case 2

A 56-year-old white female with a metastatic colon carcinoma, with multiple lesions in the liver, was treated by the IA procedure. Her primary tumor was resected in June of 1979. The complicating multiple metastatic nodules in the liver were surgically unresectable. Before being referred to us, she has had constant pain in the tumor area and had tried all forms of conventional as well as unconventional treatments with no apparent benefit. She was losing body weight, had a poor appetite, and had stopped going to work because of the associated complications. We instituted 6 IA treatments (2 treatments/week) as a first course, and 6 more as a second course, 1½ months after the first. During every IA treatment, the concentration of several plasma components decreased; among them were: total proteins, albumin, IgG, IC, IgM and IgA, α_2-macroglobulin and α_1-acid glycoprotein. There was a potentiation of white blood-cell counts and concentration of complement component C_3 increased. CEA values came down to 2550 ng/ml after the 2nd course of treatment from an initial value of 8000 ng/ml. Both phytohemagglutinin (PHA) and pokeweed mitogen (PWM)-induced blastogenic responses of peripheral blood lymphocytes (PBL) increased appreciably during the 1st course of treatment (approximately a 4-fold increase of PHA stimulatory response and a 2-fold increase in PWM stimulatory response). However, during the 2nd course of treatment, the increased level of PHA stimulatory response of PBL was not maintained. The PHA-response decreased from 4-fold increase in stimulation index (SI) after the 1st course of treatment to a 2-fold increase in SI at the end of the 2nd course of treatment. There was an appreciable increase in the percentage of rosette-forming cells (from 28% to 65%) at the end of the 2nd course of treatment. The patient showed an increased skin reactivity to a panel of recall antigens (candida, mumps, trichophyton, PPD) after the 1st course of treatment. Before the 2nd course of treatment (after an interval of 6 weeks) she became completely anergic, but she showed increased skin reactivities, again, after the 2nd course of 6 treatments. Interestingly, IgM concentration increased from 87 mg/dl to 263 mg/dl after the 1st 3 treatments; it came down to 142 mg/dl after the 5th treatment and to 117 mg/dl before the 2nd course of treatment (after an interval of treatment for 6 weeks). After the 2nd course, the concentration of IgM was elevated to 183 mg/dl. C-reactive protein (CRP) concentration in the plasma of the patient showed an increase in values after the 1st course of treatment (from 4 mg/dl to 14 mg/dl), a drop thereafter to 5 mg/dl (at the end of 6 weeks when no treatment was given), and then a rise in values to 13 mg/dl after the 2nd course of treatment was stopped. CH_{50}, which was not determined during the 1st course of treatment, was determined before and after the 2nd course of treatment. CH_{50} values increased from 35.3 units at the beginning of the 2nd course of treatment to 136.9 units after 5 subsequent treatments. The patient showed dramatic subjective improvement. A liver scan taken after the 2nd and 6th treatments showed a decrease in the tumor size. Needle biopsies taken after the 2nd and 6th treatments showed necrosis of the tumor, fibrosis, and lymphocyte infiltration. The patient felt better, had a good appetite, and gained strength. She returned to work. Her case was followed closely and she was checked every 2 to 3 weeks. Her plasma IC increased, as did the other plasma components whose concentrations were decreased after the initial course of treatment. Three months after the 2nd course of treatment, she developed ascites. Because of her disseminated disease, no further IA treatment was given. She expired. Further details of the treatment of this patient will be described elsewhere [*P. K. Ray et al.*, manuscript in preparation].

Case 3

A 50-year-old white woman with an obstructing adenocarcinoma in the sigmoid colon area was presented with a colostomy and a metastatic tumor in the liver. She was evaluated by x-rays, liver and spleen scans, bone scan, ultra-sound of the abdomen, cat scan of the brain, and other routine laboratory tests. The tumor in the sigmoid colon appeared to be resectable and removal was carried out. Two weeks after the operation she was given a series of 10 IA treatments (2 treatments/week). Liver scans taken at periodic intervals showed regression of tumor in the liver. All of the immunological parameters studied in the case of patient nr. 2 were repeated during the course of the treatment of this patient. In general, the data for all of the parameters tested showed similar trends of increase and/ or decrease for the various blood components. Her CEA values came down (from 115 ng/ml to 80 ng/ml) after 5 treatments, as did her IgG and IC values. At the completion of her last treatment, she underwent closure of her colostomy. After two months, her CEA values showed an increase. Her liver scan and immunological data did not show much of a change, although she showed an increase in IgG and immune complex concentrations. There was also an increase in the concentration of her CEA values. Considering this, she was called back for a further course of 4 IA treatments. The liver scans taken before the additional treatments, and at the end of them were compared. They showed appreciable reduction of the tumor volume. The patient was released from the hospital and continued to be followed. Since then she has received periodic IA treatments and has been living a normal life. As of this writing, she is now 400 days post diagnosis of her colon neoplasm. The details of treatment will be published elsewhere [P. K. Ray et al., manuscript in preparation].

Case 4

A 58-year-old white male was presented in a Chicago hospital in August 1980 with a history, over several months, of decreasing caliber of stool. Approximately 10 days prior to admission he became unable to pass any stool. Lower GI x-rays showed a complete obstruction. Flexible sigmoidoscopy was performed on the day of operation; the operator was unable to pass the scope beyond 22 cms, due to the obstruction. A transverse colostomy was made. Exploration of the abdominal cavity by hand showed the liver extensively infiltrated with metastatic disease and there was penetration into the anterior abdominal wall. There were also several other implants in the anterior abdominal wall. There was a mass in the colon at the level of the pelvic brim. There were also multiple metastatic implants on the mesentery. At that time only a colostomy was done.

The patient was presented at the Medical College of Pennsylvania in January 1981, with his colostomy still functioning. After he was thoroughly evaluated the primary tumor in his lower GI tract was removed along with several masses from the abdominal wall. After two weeks, the patient was given 4 IA treatments (2 treatments/week). He showed changes similar to those described for the other patients in the immune components of his blood. A week later, he received 2 more IA treatments, and his colostomy was closed. He was released from the hospital and is still being followed. At the time of writing this paper (3 months past IA treatment), he is doing well, with no complications or problems. He showed significant subjective and objective improvement as a result of the treatment. He has a good appetite and has gained weight. The details of the treatment of this patient will be published elsewhere [*P. K. Ray et al.*, manuscript in preparation].

Case 5

In 1980, this 82-year-old white male was presented to his physician at the Medical College of Pennsylvania for an obstruction in his colon, which was surgically corrected. In June 1981, he was presented again with an enlarged liver filled with metastatic tumor. He was given 4 IA treatments (2 treatments/week). He showed both subjective and objective improvements. A liver scan before treatment showed a homogeneous area; after IA treatment, it looked smaller in shape, somewhat nonhomogeneous, and fragmented in appearance. The patient felt better and was released from the hospital. At the time of this writing (5½ months after IA treatment), he is doing well, with no complaints.

Discussion

It appears from: (1) those experiences in treating human cancer patients which we have described here, (2) others which will be described elsewhere (our experiences in treating bronchogenic carcinoma, glioma, and astrocytoma patients, also patients with other types of malignancies) and (3) those which have been published previously [28, 32–34], that plasma adsorption with SPA can augment the immunological reactivities of the tumor host. We think that these increased immune reactivities are possibly directed against tumor growth so that either: (a) the growth of tumors is arrested, and/or (b) the tumors undergo regression. Histopathological data indicate increased fibrosis and necrosis in the tumor, neovascularization, and lymphocyte infiltration. Radiological scans show decrease in the size of the tumor during the course of IA treatment. Some of our patients, whose treatment was discontinued, had a recurrence of their tumors. However, by careful follow-up and periodic testing and repetition of the IA treatments, we have been able to maintain the patient in reasonably good health; in one case for more than 400 days from the time her disease was discovered (primary colon carcinoma with liver metastases). Several other patients are under close observation; however, no definitive assessment can be made as yet regarding their long-term clinical status. In any event, all of these patients who: (1) had a considerable amount of tumor load; (2) had metastasized tumors; or (3) experienced failures of other forms of treatment, showed significant subjective and some positive objective improvement following IA treatments. We do not know exactly: (1) where this form of treatment may find its best use; (2) what type(s) of tumor may respond best; (3) if the treatment may be able to offer better therapeutic benefit in patients with a smaller tumor load, compared to far advanced cases; (4) if the previous treatments may have an influence on the outcome of the treatment; (5) if the initial clinical status of the patient and the existing immunological profile may reflect upon the outcome of the treatment; or (6) if other types of therapy along with IA treatment may be more advantageous than IA alone. We are investigating these and other aspects of the treatment extensively. In future reports we hope to have resolved more of the questions.

The exact mechanism, by which IA treatment can induce tumoricidal reactions, is not known. Animal data obtained in our laboratory have indicated that killer-cell activity and antibody-dependent cell-mediated cytotoxicity (ADCC) was significantly increased in the peripheral blood lymphocytes from immunoadsorbed rats [27, 29, 31] showing tumor regression. We have also observed that in plasma of animals undergoing IA treatment, cytotoxic antibody activity can be demonstrated [27, 29, 31]. However, sham-treated controls do not show such a response. Further, plasma from sham-treated controls showed blocking activity against PBL *in vitro,* whereas the plasma from the treated animals showed ADCC reaction and no blocking effect. We have observed similar potentiation of killer-cell activity and ADCC reaction using PBL and plasma from one of our patients (Case nr. 4) [32]. Thus it appears that immunologically similar reactions can be induced in both tumor-bearing animals and in human cancer patients subsequent to IA treatment. The increased antibody activity in the immunoadsorbed tumor-hosts is a consistent observation in our laboratory. Potentiation of T- and B-cell response, increased rosette (EA rosette)-forming ability of T-lymphocytes, increased skin reactivity, increased CH_{50}, and elevated level of IgM concentrations are almost always correlated with the therapeutic improvement of the tumor host and a decrease in the concentration of immune complexes, IgG, Ca, and cold agglutinin. The detailed results of these mechanistic studies await publication.

The future of the IA treatment is uncertain, but it has shown results that are sufficiently promising to justify extensive investigation; either to confirm or to negate these initial observations.

Acknowledgment

The authors gratefully acknowledge financial assistance received from R. J. Reynolds Industries, Inc., Fannie E. Ripple Foundation, and W. W. Smith Charitable Trust in support of this investigation.

References

1   Old, L. J.; Boyse, E. A.: Immunology of experimental tumors. Annu. Rev. Med. *15:* 167 (1964).
2   Sjogren, H. O.: Transplantation methods as a tool for detection of tumor-specific antigens. Prog. exp. Tumor Res. *6:* 289 (1965).
3   Rosenau, W.; Morton, D. L.: Tumor-specific inhibition of growth of methylcholanthrene-induced sarcomas *in vivo* and *in vitro* by sensitized isologous lymphoid cells. J. natn. Cancer Inst. *36:* 825 (1966).
4   Hellstrom, I.; Hellstrom, K. E.; Pierce, G. E.: *In vitro* studies of immune reactions against autochthonous and synergic mouse tumor by methylcholanthrene and plastic discs. Int. J. Cancer *3:* 467 (1968).
5   Ray, P. K.; Saha, S.: Development of humoral and cellular tumor growth-enhancing factors may depend on the concentration of tumor antigen present. J. natn. Cancer Inst. (communicated).
6   Raychaudhuri, S.; Ray, P. K.; Bassett, J. G.; Cooper, D. R.: High-dose antigen-induced suppressor generation in normal and tumor-bearing hosts. Fed. Proc. *39* (3): 696 (1980).
7   Hellstrom, I.; Hellstrom, K. E.: Studies on cellular immunity and its serum-mediated inhibition in Moloney virus-induced mouse sarcomas. Int. J. Cancer *4:* 587 (1969).
8   Sjogren, H. O.; Hellstrom, I.; Bansal, S. C.; Hellstrom, K. E.: Suggestive evidence that the 'blocking antibodies' of tumor-bearing individuals may be antigen-antibody complexes. Proc. natn. Acad. Sci. USA *68:* 1372 (1971).
9   Alexander, P.: Escape from immune destruction by the host through shedding of surface antigens: Is this a characteristic shared by malignant and embryonic cells? Cancer Res. *34:* 2077 (1974).
10 Kirchner, H.; Chused, T. M.; Herberman, R. B.; Holden, H. T.; Lavrin, D. H.: Evidence of suppressor-cell activity in spleens of mice bearing primary tumors induced by Moloney sarcoma virus. J. exp. Med. *139:* 1473 (1974).
11 Greene, M. I.; Fuzimoto, S.; Sehon, A. H.: Regulation of the immune response to tumor antigens. III. Characterization of thymic suppressor factor (3) produced by tumor-bearing hosts. J. Immun. *119:* 757 (1977).
12 Ankerest, J.: Demonstration and identification of cytotoxic antibodies and antibodies blocking的 cell-mediated antitumor immunity against adenoviurs-12-induced tumors. Cancer Res. *31:* 997 (1971).
13 Sakesla, E.; Pentinnen, K.; Pirohonen, S.: Non-specific blocking of human ovarian carcinoma-associated cellular cytotoxicity *in vitro*. Scand. J. Immunol. *3:* 781 (1974).
14 Witz, I. P.: Biological significance of tumor-bound immunoglobulins. Curr. Top. Microbiol. Immunol. *61:* 151 (1973).

15 Baldwin, R. W.; Price, M. R.; Robins, R. A.: Blocking of lymphocyte-mediated cytotoxicity for rat hepatoma cells by specific antigen-antibody complexes. Nature new Biol. *238:* 185 (1972).

16 Israel, L.; Edelstein, R.; Mannoni, P.: Plasmapheresis in patients with disseminated cancer: Clinical results and correlation with changes in serum protein. The concept of non-specific blocking factors. Cancer *40:* 3146 (1977).

17 Sulica, A.; Kaly, M.; Gherman, M.; Ghetie, V.; Sjoquist, J.: Arming of lymphoid cells by IgG antibodies treated with protein-A from *Staphylococcus aureus.* Scand. J. Immunol. *5:* 1102 (1976).

18 Voisin, G. A.: Immunity and tolerance: A unified concept. Cell Immunol. *2:* 670 (1971).

19 Baldwin, R. W.; Embuton, M. J.; Price, M. R.; Robins, A.: Immunity in the tumor-bearing host and its modification by serum factors. Cancer *34:* 1452 (1974).

20 Kerbel, R. S.; Davies, A. J. S.: The possible biological significance of Fc-receptors on mammalian lymphocytes and tumor cells. Cell *3:* 105 (1974).

21 Gershon, R. K.; Mokyr, M. B.; Mitchell, M. S.: Activation of suppressor T-cells by tumor cells and specific antibody. Nature *250:* 594 (1974).

22 Oldstone, M. B. A.; Tishow, A.: Active thymus-derived suppressor lymphocytes in human cord blood. Nature *269:* 333 (1977).

23 Peter, H. H.; Pavie-Fischer, J.; Fridman, W. H.; Aubert, C.; Cesarini, J. P.; Roubin, R.; Kouridsky, F. M.: Cell-mediated cytotoxicity *in vitro* of human lymphocytes against a tissue culture melanoma cell line (IgR3). J. Immun. *115:* 539 (1975).

24 Cowan, F. M.; Klein, D. L.; Armstrong, G. R.; Pearson, J. W.: Neutralization of immune complex inhibition of antibody-dependent cellular cytotoxicity *in vitro* by *Staphylococcus aureus* protein A. Biomed. *30:* 23 (1979).

25 Bansal, S. C.; Bansal, B. R.; Boland, J. P.: Blocking and unblocking factors in neoplasms. Curr. Top. Microbiol. Immunol. *75:* 45 (1976).

26 Wright, P. W.; Hellstrom, K. E.; Hellstrom, I.: Serotherapy of malignant disease. Med. Clins N. Am. *60:* 607 (1976).

27 Ray, P. K.; Cooper, D. R.; Bassett, J. G.; Mark, R.: Antitumor effect of *Staphylococcus aureus* organisms. Fed. Proc. *38* (3): 1089 (1979).

28 Ray, P. K.; Idiculla, A.; Rhoads, J. E., Jr.; Mark, R.; Besa, E.; Thomas, H.; Bassett, J. G.; Cooper, D. R.: Extracorporeal immunoadsorption of pathologic plasma immunoglobulin-G or its complexes. A novel approach for their selective removal from the plasma. In: Proceedings of the First Annual Apheresis Symposium: Current Concepts and Future Trends, pp. 203–215 (Chicago 1979).

29 Ray, P. K.; Idiculla, A.; Rhoads, J. E., Jr.; Mark, R.; Bassett, J. G.; Cooper, D. R.: Immunoadsorption of blocking immune complexes using *Staphylococcus aureus* protein-A column – A novel approach for immunotherapy of cancer. Fourth Intl. Congress of Immunology. 10. 5. 57 (Paris, July 1980).

30 Ray, P. K.; Mohammed, J.; Raychaudhuri, S.; Bassett, J. G.; Cooper, D. R.: Growth inhibition of rat primary mammary adenocarcinomas by immunoadsorption of blocking immune complexes. Fourth Intl. Congress of Immunology. 10. 7. 25 (Paris, July 1980).

31 Ray, P. K.; Raychaudhuri, S.; Mark, R.; Bassett, J. G.; Cooper, D. R.: Growth inhibition of DMBA-induced rat mammary adenocarcinomas by *ex vivo* immunoadsorption of plasma with protein-A containing *Staphylococcus aureus.* Proc. Amer. Ass. Cancer Res. *72:* 1124 (1981).

32 Ray, P. K.; Idiculla, A.; Clarke, L.; Rhoads, J. E., Jr.; Mark, R.; Bassett, J. G.; Cooper, D. R.: Immunoadsorption of IgG and/or its complexes from colon carcinoma patients-- An adjunct therapy for cancer. Proc. Intl. Conf. Adjuvant Therapy of Cancer, p. 29 (Tucson, Arizona, March 1981).

33   Ray, P. K.; McLaughlin, D.; Mohammed, J.; Idiculla, A.; Rhoads, J. E., Jr.; Mark, R.;
       Bassett, J. G.; Cooper, D. R.: *Ex vivo* immunoadsorption of IgG or its complexes--A
       new modality of cancer treatment. In: Serrou, Rosenfeld (eds.), Immune complexes
       and Plasma Exchanges in Cancer Patients, pp. 197–207 (Elsevier/North Holland
       Biomedical Press, Amsterdam 1981).
34   Ray, P. K.; Idiculla, A.; Mark, R.; Rhoads, J. E., Jr.; Thomas, H.; Bassett, J. G.;
       Cooper, D. R.: Extracorporeal immunoadsorption of plasma from a metastatic colon
       carcinoma patient by protein A-containing non-viable *Staphylococcus aureus*. Clinical,
       biochemical, serological, and histological evaluation of the patient's response. Cancer
       (in press, 1981).
35   Bansal, S. C.; Bansal, B. R.; Thomas, H. L.: *Ex vivo* removal of serum-IgG in a patient
       with colon carcinoma. Cancer *43:* 1 (1978).
36   Isbister, W. H.; Noonan, F. P.; Halliday, W. J.: Human thoracic duct cannulation.
       Manipulation of tumor-specific blocking factors in a patient with malignant melanoma.
       Cancer *35:* 1465 (1975).
37   Sjoquist, J.: Structure and immunology of protein-A. In: Jelijaszewcz, Hryniewicz
       (eds.), Staphylococci and Streptococcal Infections, pp. 83–92 (S. Karger, Basel 1973).
38   McDougal, J. S.; Redecha, P. B.; Inman, R. D.; Christian, C. L.: Binding of immuno-
       globulin-G aggregates and immune complexes in human sera to staphylococci contain-
       ing protein-A. J. clin. Invest. *63:* 627 (1979).
39   Kessler, S. W.: Rapid isolation of antigens from cells with a staphylococcal protein-A
       antibody adsorbent: Parameters of the interaction of antibody-antigen complexes with
       protein-A. J. Immun. *115:* 1617 (1975).
40   Ray, P. K.; Besa, E.; Idiculla, A.; Rhoads, J. E., Jr.; Bassett, J. G.; Cooper, D. R.:
       Efficient removal of abnormal immunoglobulin-G from the plasma of a multiple
       myeloma patient – Description of a new method for treatment of the hyperviscosity
       syndrome. Cancer *45:* 2633 (1980).
41   Ray, P. K.; Idiculla, A.; Rhoads, J. E., Jr.; Besa, E.; Bassett, J. G.; Cooper, D. R.:
       Extracorporeal immunoadsorption of myeloma-IgG and autoimmune antibodies – A
       clinically feasible modality of treatment. Clin. exp. Immunol. *42:* 308 (1980).
42   Ray, P. K.; Idiculla, A.; Rhoads, J. E., Jr.; Besa, E.; Bassett, J. G.; Cooper, D. R.:
       Immunoadsorption of IgG-molecules from the plasma of multiple myeloma and auto-
       immune hemolytic anemia patients. Plasma Ther. *1:* 11 (1980).

Dr. P. K. Ray, Departments of Surgery and Microbiology, The Medical College of Pennsylvania and Hospital, 3300 Henry Avenue, USA-Philadelphia, PA 19129

Absorption of Human Plasma on Protein A-Sepharose: Effects on in Vitro Parameters of Tumor Immunity[1]

H. O. Sjögren, A. Wallmark, P. Flodgren, A. Grubb, B. Husberg, T. Lindholm, C. Lindström, H. Thysell

The Wallenberg Laboratory, Department of Oncology and Department of Nephrology, University of Lund, Sweden
Department of Clinical Chemistry, Department of Surgery, and Department of Pathology, Malmö General Hospital, Sweden

Introduction

There are several lines of evidence indicating that the appearance of serum-blocking factors (SBF) in tumor patients inhibit the potency of antitumor-cellular immunity in vivo [1, 2, 3]. These blocking factors include several different entities among which some exert a blocking that is specific for antitumor immunity and others that are generally suppressive. Examples of the former type are the circulating complexes of tumor antigens and antitumor antibodies [4] and some immunoglobulin subclasses which cannot activate the complement cascade and which do not mediate ADCC. It is of great principal interest to be able to eliminate these blocking factors selectively and to study whether or not this may have an immunotherapeutical effect. The usefulness of Staph. aureus, Cowan I, which contains protein A, was suggested for this purpose by the investigations of *Steele et al.* [5]. Absorption of rat colon carcinoma bearer's sera with these bacteria removed the serum-blocking activity as assayed in

[1] Supported by grants from the Swedish Cancer Society, John and Augusta Persson's Foundation, and the Medical Faculty, University of Lund, Sweden. The skillful technical assistance of *Ms. Maria Lassen, Ms. Ingar Nilsson,* and *Ms. Barbro Sjögren* is gratefully acknowledged as is the technical support of Gambro AB in connection with the plasma absorption procedures.

vitro and lead to the detectability of complement-dependent cytotoxic antibodies previously not demonstrable. Similar absorption of sera from human cancer patients confirmed the elimination of serum-blocking factors [6]. *Bansal et al.* [7] developed an extracorporeal system in dogs which allowed the absorption of large plasma volumes on large quantitities of heat-inactivated, formaline-stabilized Staph. aureus. Repeated absorptions of this kind in dogs with spontaneous malignancies indicated tumor-inhibitory effects [8]. A similar procedure with batch absorption of plasma in leukemic cats clearly indicated a therapeutic effect [9].

Extracorporeal plasma absorption on two human patients with recurrent adenocarcinoma of the colon has also been reported [8, 10]. The patients were subjected to 19 and 8 procedures respectively and therapeutical effects were recorded.

It has been implied that the absorption by Staph. aureus, Cowan I is due to immunoglobulin absorption on protein A. On that basis we have studied the effects of plasma absorption in protein A-Sepharose columns (Pharmacia Fine Chemicals and Gambro AB, Sweden). The absorption procedure was tolerated well by dogs with and without spontaneous neoplasms. A total of 35 absorptions were subsequently performed in four human patients with advanced stages of colon carcinoma and kidney carcinoma.

We describe here the approach taken to analyze the possible changes in the patients' immunity to their own tumors and report studies applied to two patients.

Results

There are numerous indications for the existence of tissue type-specific antigens in human tumors against which the tumor patients mount immune responses [1, 11, 12]. This immunity can often be found in a fairly large proportion of the patients and the specificity can be proven by studies of relatively large groups of patients. However, when the immunity of an individual patient is to be analyzed, the tumor specificity of the immune responses becomes a major problem, especially when allogeneic target cells are used. Therefore, we have exclusively used autochthonous neoplastic and non-neoplastic cells as targets to avoid reactions to irrelevant antigens. However, even when autochthonous target cells are used, the presence of spontaneously cytotoxic lymphocytes (NK-cells) and monocytes makes it often difficult to evaluate specific cellular tumor immunity. It is of great importance to be able to distinguish clearly between the effects of monocytes, NK-cells, K-cells, and T-killer cells. The availibility of techniques to separate these various effector cells is therefore essential for a detailed analysis. Also it is of great importance for serological analysis to have the autochthonous cells available.

Our approach to the separation problem is to use a 3-step procedure as summarized in table I. Mononuclear blood cells are isolated by the Ficoll-Isopaque centrifugation technique [13]. Monocytes are eliminated by sedimentation at unit gravity. Finally, K- and NK-cells are isolated together, and separated from most of the other lymphocytes by using a two-phase dextran-PEG system which has been modified from what was previously described [14, 15]. The distribution of lymphocytes in this two-phase system is illustrated in figure 1. Most cells are recovered in the left part of the CCD curve, separate from a minority of cells which distribute into fractions 75–110. The NK-activity, assayed on sensitive K562 target cells, is enriched in the latter fractions (L8) with only minor activities demonstrable in the other fractions (fig. 2).

Immunological studies was performed on two patients subjected to plasma absorption of protein A-Sepharose. Plasma was separated by an Aminco cell centrifuge (American Instrument Co.) and passed through one or two columns containing a total of 140–280 ml of protein A-Sepharose (SpA) (Pharmacia Fine Chemicals) which have a total binding capacity of approximately 3.5–7.0 g of IgG. The absorbed plasma was reinfused into the patient after passing through a sterile filter.

A 41-year-old female, with a colonic carcinoma showing local recurrent growth and distant metastases to liver and lung, did not respond to

Table I. Lymphocyte separation for immunological analysis

Technique	Purpose
Ficoll-Isopaque centrifugation	Isolation of mononuclear cells
Sedimentation at 1×g in a Percoll gradient followed by elimination of cells adherent to plastic	Isolation of (1) lymphocytes free of monocytes, (2) large lymphocytes separate from small lymphocytes, (3) monocyte-enriched cells
Dextran-PEG two-phase separation of lymphocytes with counter-current distribution	Enrichment of NK- and K-cells, separate from cells mediating cytotoxicity selective for tumor cells

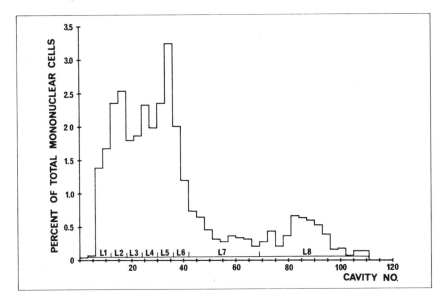

Fig. 1. Mononuclear blood cells, obtained from a colonic carcinoma patient, were fractionated in a dextran-PEG two-phase system in a counter-current distribution (CCD) apparatus [17]. The phase system was composed of 5% dextran T 500, 4% polyethylene glycol 6000, 0.06 M, sodium phosphate buffer pH 7.4, 0.05 M sodium chloride, and 5% heat-inactivated fetal calf serum. The phases were mixed and equilibrated in a separator funnel at 4°C over night. The PEG top phase and the dextran bottom phase were then separated and the phases were loaded into an automatic CCD apparatus with circular plates [17] with 120 cavities and the bottom plate capacity of .67 ml per cavity. The apparatus was run at +4°C and cells collected as previously described [14]. After determining the cell distribution by counting in an automatic cell counter (Coulter Counter Corp.), fractions were pooled (L1–L8) and assayed in vitro.

chemotherapy. She was subjected to 15 absorption procedures with no acute adverse reactions. No conclusive therapeutic effect was demonstrated at the time of immunological analysis.

Peripheral blood cells were obtained before absorption treatment was initiated and after the 7th procedure. They were separated by the described 3-step procedure. After separation at unit gravity (fig. 3), monocyte-depleted fractions were pooled (= L1), monocyte-enriched fractions (above 40% monocytes) were pooled (= L3), and the pool of other fractions (= L2) was incubated for one hour in plastic tissue culture bottles to remove adherent cells. Cells corresponding to pool L1 were further fractionated in a dextran-PEG two-phase system (fig. 4). An increased proportion of the cells was recovered to the right of the distribution as compared to the proportion recovered just before the first plasma absorption was performed. Various fractions were tested for selective cytotoxicity to cultured autochthonous tumor cells and compared with cytotoxicity to normal fibroblasts. They were simultaneously evaluated for K- and NK-activity.

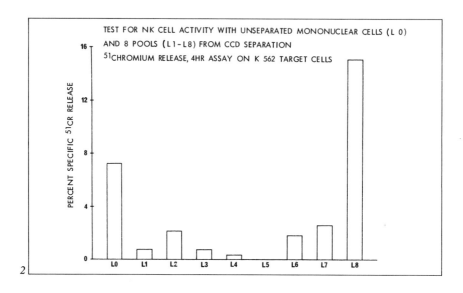

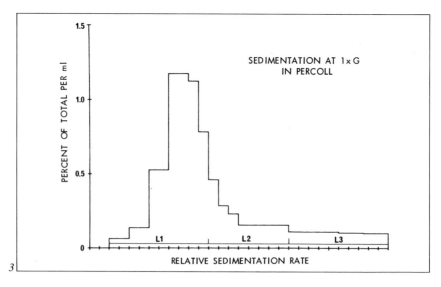

Figure 5 illustrates the selective cytotoxicity recorded against autochthonous tumor cells at the 10:1 ratio with blood cells obtained after the 7th absorption procedure. The first two CCD fractions (L4 and L5) showed a clear-cut selective effect on the tumor cells, while the unseparated mononuclear cells had no such effect. The other ratios tested (20:1 and 40:1) showed the same pattern with selective effects demonstrated in L4 and L5 (not illustrated). The test performed before initiation of absorption treatment also demonstrated selective cytotoxicity to the corresponding CCD fractions but only at an E/T ratio of 80:1 and showed no selective effect on unseparated cells.

Simultaneously performed tests demonstrated a high K- and a low NK-activity before treatment. After 7 plasma absorptions the K-cell activity became even higher while the NK-activity remained low, even in fractions in which it was relatively enriched (fig. 6).

Tests for complement-dependent serum cytotoxicity remained negative through out the treatment period. Assays for ADCC with the patient's sera on autochthonous target cells, using rat spleen cells as a

---

◁   *Fig. 2.* Various fractions of mononuclear blood cells obtained from a female colonic carcinoma patient who was later subjected to plasma absorption were tested for NK-cell activity. The K562 cell line [18, 19] was used as a sensitive target for NK-cells in a 4 h ^{51}Chromium release assay [15]. K562 cells were labeled with sodium chromate (^{51}Cr) and mixb with the various lymphocyte fractions in an effector to target (E/T) ratio of 20:1. The results of three lower ratios are not presented. Three parallells were used per fraction. Released ^{51}Cr activity above spontaneous release (in absence of lymphocytes) was calculated. Specific release was calculated as

$$\frac{\text{(experimental release} - \text{spontaneous release)} \times 100}{\text{maximum releasable (zapoglobin)} - \text{spontaneous release}}$$

The spread was small and generally a specific release of 1–2 % was statistically significant according to Student's t-test.

Fig. 3. Ficoll-Isopaque separated mononuclear blood cells were obtained from a colonic carcinoma patient subjected to 7 SpA-Sepharose plasma absorptions. The cells were washed in PBS and placed at +4°C on a Percoll gradient (400 ml, density 1.005–1.020 g/ml) containing 5% fetal calf serum in a chamber designed according to *Bont et al.* [20]. After sedimentation for two hours at 1×g, fractions of 10 to 20 ml were removed from the visible lymphocyte band and downwards. The number of cells per fraction was counted (Coulter Counter Corp.) and the size distribution analyzed (C1000, Multi Channel Analyzer) as a rapid way of determining the proportion of monocytes. Fractions depleted of monocytes were pooled (L1), fractions containing more than 40% monocytes were similarly pooled (L3), and a pool of the remaining fractions (L2) was incubated for one hour in plastic tissue culture bottles to remove adherent cells. Pool L1 cells were further separated in the dextran-PEG two-phase system (fig. 4), while the other two pools were stored for 20 h at +4°C until being assayed.

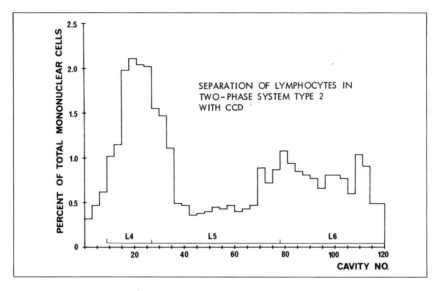

Fig. 4. Monocyte-depleted fractions of mononuclear blood cells were obtained from a colonic carcinoma patient, who had been subjected to 7 plasma absorptions, were subjected to counter-current distribution (L1 of fig. 3). The fractions were pooled to give L4, L5, and L6 as indicated. These pools were assayed for cytotoxicity.

Fig. 5. Selective lymphocyte cytotoxicity was tested against autochthonous tumor cells ▷ in a female colonic carcinoma patient who was subjected to 7 plasma absorptions on SpA-Sepharose. Various fractions of mononuclear blood cells were separated (A) by sedimentation at $1 \times g$, (L0–L3 of fig. 3); and (B) by CCD (L4, L5, L6 of fig. 4) were assayed. Monolayer cultures of the patient's own tumor cells and skin fibroblasts were used as targets after being established and frozen in liquid nitrogen before treatment of the patient had been initiated. The cells were allowed to attach to the flat bottoms of glass ampoules (Flow Laboratories) by overnight incubation at 37°C. Attached cells were labeled with sodium chromate (^{51}Cr) as previously described [15]. Lymphocytes suspended in 0.2 ml of RPMI 1640 medium supplemented with 5% fetal calf serum and 10 mmol Hepes were added in ratios from 10:1 to 80:1 (ratio 10:1 presented in this diagram). After incubation for 20 h at 37°C the tubes were centrifuged and the radioactivity of samples of the supernatants were determined in a Gamma Counter (Beckman 310). Spontaneous release was estimated in the absence of effector cells and the maxium releasable isotope was estimated in tubes with addition of zapoglobin in destilled water. The percentage of specific release was calculated as

$$\frac{\text{release with lymphocytes} - \text{spontaneous release}}{\text{maximum releasable} - \text{spontaneous release}} \times 100\%.$$

The significance of results was estimated by Student's t-test. Approximately 3% release was significant on at least the 5% level. Differences between effects on tumor and fibroblast target cells are shaded when the effect on tumor is larger.

source of K-effector cells with relatively low NK-activity, did not reveal any humoral antibodies with tumor specificity. Low pH eluates from the SpA-Sepharose columns did not show any detectable antitumor-antibody activity through these two assays.

Immunological analysis was also performed before and after one plasma-absorption procedure on SpA-Sepharose of a 57-year-old male patient with multiple metastases of a kidney carcinoma. Ficoll-Isopaque separated mononuclear cells and three CCD fractions, one of which (fraction 3) was enriched with regard to NK-activity, were tested for cytotoxicity to autochthonous tumor cells and fibroblasts (table II). The two CCD

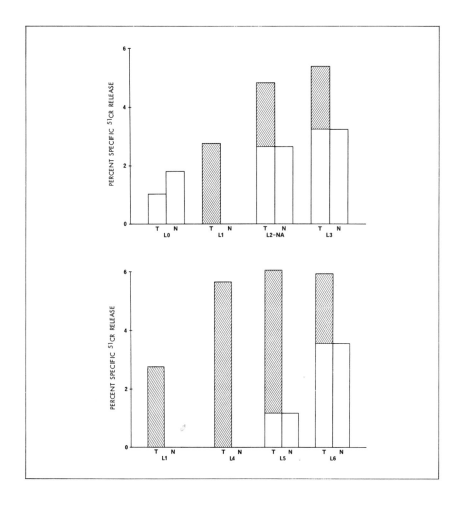

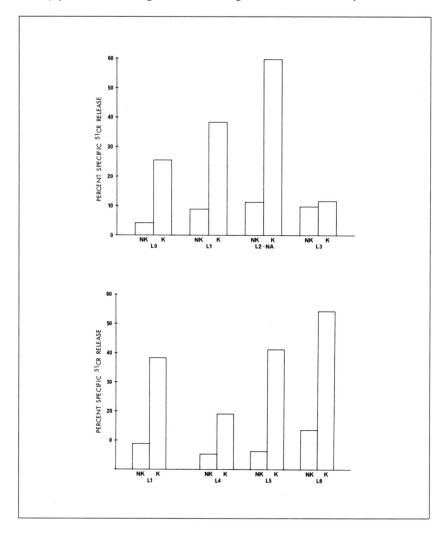

Fig. 6. Tests for K and NK cell activity were performed on various fractions of mono-nuclear blood cells separated (A) by sedimentation at $1 \times g$ (L0–L3 of text fig. 3) and (B) by CCD (L4–L6, fig. 4) from a female colonic carcinoma patient who was subjected to 7 plasma absorptions on SpA-Sepharose. NK-cell activity was assayed at 4 E/T ratios as previously described (fig. 2). Ratio 8:1 is presented in this diagram. K-cell activity was determined as previously described [15] using NK-resistant rat thymocytes preincubated with an appropriate rabbit antibody as targets. At least 3 E/T ratios were tested of which only ratio 8:1 is presented. The various effector cells were not cytotoxic in absence of the antiserum, nor did the antiserum cause any cytolysis in absence of effector cells.

Table II. Test for lymphocyte cytotoxicity in a kidney carcinoma patient after one plasma absorption with SpA-Sepharose

Lymphocyte fraction		Ratio	Percent specific ^{51}Cr release	
		E/T	Autochthonous tumor cells	Autochthonous fibroblasts
Ficoll-Isopaque separated mononuclear cells		80:1	10.6 p < 0.05	15.2 p < 0.05
		40:1	0.8	11.7 p < 0.05
		20:1	2.1	3.8
		10:1	3.4	7.7
Monocyte-depleted mononuclear cells separated by CCD	Fraction 1	80:1	6.8 p < 0.05	0 (−2.4)
		40:1	0.4	0 (−1.8)
		20:1	5.6	0 (−3.5)
		10:1	0 (−1.5)	0 (−2.6)
	Fraction 2	80:1	–	–
		40:1	10.8 p < 0.05	0 (−6.2)
		20:1	0.9	0 (−4.6)
		10:1	2.9	0 (−5.7)
	Fraction 3	80:1	–	–
		40:1	3.5	0.2
		20:1	0.1	3.2
		10:1	2.4	5.3

fractions with minimal NK-activity had a selective effect on the tumor cells, while the unseparated mononuclear cells showed cytotoxicity against both target cell types, of which the fibroblasts were most sensitive.

Tests for complement-dependent cytotoxicity showed that this patient had antibodies with selective effect on the autochthonous tumor cells before the patient was subjected to plasma absorption (table III). This activity increased significantly when tested 9 days after the treatment. Antibodies with a selective effect on autochthonous tumor cells were also demonstrated in tests for ADCC using BN rat lymphocyte effector cells. Also this activity increased in the sample obtained after the patient was treated. Selective complement-dependent cytotoxicity against auto-chthonous tumor cells was also demonstrated in low pH eluates from the SpA-Sepharose columns used for absorption (table IV).

Conclusions

Absorption of plasma by protein A-Sepharose columns is technically feasable. The columns can be reused for the same patient 15 times or more

Table III. A kidney carcinoma patient tested for complement dependent cytolysis[1] before and after one plasma absorption with SpA-Sepharose

Time of serum sample	Dilution	Percent specific ^{51}Cr release	
		Autochthonous tumor cells	Autochthonous fibroblasts
26 days before treatment	1:10	9.2 p < 0.001	0 (−0.6)
	1:20	8.1 p < 0.001	0 (−1.8)
	1:40	0.7	0 (−1.9)
Immediately before treatment	1:10	16.1 p < 0.001	0 (−1.7)
	1:20	4.1 p < 0.01	0 (−0.8)
	1:40	0.4	0 (−1.7)
9 days after treatment	$1:10^2$	56.2 p < 0.001	0.3
	1:20	43.7 p < 0.001	0 (−0.2)
	1:40	18.2 p < 0.001	0 (−0.1)
	1:80	7.4 p < 0.001	0 (−0.7)
	1:160	2.7	1.1

[1] All serum samples were stored frozen at −20°C until assayed simultaneously against cultured autochthonous tumor cells and fibroblasts. The cells were allowed to attach to the flat bottom surfaces of glass ampoules by overnight incubation at 37°C. The tubes were labelled with ^{51}Cr as previously described [15]. After washing the attached cells, serum dilutions were added to duplicate tubes (0.2 ml/tube) and incubated for 30 min. Serum was aspirated and rabbit complement added and incubated for 2 h, after which the tubes were centrifugated and the radioactivity of samples of supernatants were estimated in a Gamma Counter (Beckman 310).

[2] Serum dilution 1:10 with inactivated complement had no cytolytic effect (−0.1%) on the autochthonous tumor cells.

if absorbed material is eluted at low pH after each absorption procedure. An intentional overloading of the columns, by passing up to 3 l of plasma through columns which have the capacity to absorb the IgG of 0.5–1.0 l of plasma (7 g IgG), is being performed with the aim to achieve a selective removal of molecules which have the strongest binding to protein A. Immune complexes are believed to bind stronger than free IgG, although detailed analysis of human immune complexes are still lacking. It is also likely that some IgG subclasses bind stronger than others [16], but the functional results of selective absorption of certain IgG subclasses still remains to be elucidated.

We have demonstrated that passing heparinized plasma through SpA-Sepharose columns activates a large part of the C3 into C3b. Mixing of heparinized plasma with Staph. aureus, Cowan I also activates a major

Table IV. Tests were performed for selective complement-dependent cytotoxicity to autochthonous tumor cells in low pH eluates from SpA-Sepharose which had been for plasma absorption in a male kidney carcinoma patient

Elution	Dilution[1]	Percent specific ^{51}Cr release[2]	
pH	Relative to passed plasma	Autochthonous tumor cells	Autochthonous fibroblasts
4.5	3:1	54.9***	0 (−0.7)
	3:1[3]	0 (−3.6)	0 (−1.8)
	1:1	24.6***	0 (−0.1)
	1:3	0 (−2.0)	0
	1:10	0 (−1.9)	0 (−0.5)
	1:30	0 (−2.9)	−
4.0	3:1	68.4***	1.1
	3:1[3]	0 (−4.3)	0 (−1.7)
	1:1	42.1***	0 (−0.9)
	1:3	23.2***	0 (−0.2)
	1:10	2.0	0 (−2.2)
	1:10[3]	0 (−4.8)	0 (−3.5)
	1:30	0 (−3.6)	−
3.0	10:1	59.0***	0 (−0.9)
	3:1	39.5***	0 (−2.4)
	3:1[3]	0 (−3.4)	0 (−2.8)
	1:1	17.8***	0 (−2.4)
	1:3	0 (−0.6)	0 (−1.0)
	1:10	0 (−3.2)	0 (−1.0)
	1:30	0 (−3.4)	−

[1] Eluates were diluted in relation to the total volume of plasma passed through the column. Normal human serum was added to the various dilutions to a final concentration of 1:20. The same normal serum was included in the test. The difference in ^{51}Cr release with active versus inactivated complement was for this normal serum 1.8% on tumor cells and 2.1% on fibroblasts.

[2] Specific ^{51}Cr release was calculated as

$$\frac{\% \text{ release with test sample} - \% \text{ release with normal serum}}{\% \text{ maximum release} - \% \text{ release with normal serum}} \times 100\%$$

Significance was calculated according to the Student's t-test and is indicated as ***: p < 0.001; **: p < 0.01; *: p < 0.05.

[3] Inactivated complement was used (incubation for 30 min at 56°C).

part of the C3. Detectable C3 activation does not occur on SpA-Sepharose in the presence of citrate.

By using the described lymphocyte separation procedure it appears to be possible to detect selective lymphocyte cytotoxicity for the autochthonous tumor cells. This may make it possible to monitor the effects on tumor immunity with this plasma-absorption technique, which will be of great importance in clarifying the mechanisms of possible therapeutic effects with this or similar procedures.

There was a significant increase in the titer of antibodies-mediating complement-dependent cytolysis and ADCC in one of the patients studied. In the other patient no humoral antibodies were detected but there were indications of an increased level of selective lymphocyte cytotoxicity against autochthonous tumor cells, and of K-cell activity. There was no evidence of stimulated NK-cell activity in either patient.

References

1   Hellström, K. E.; Hellström, I.: Lymphocyte-mediated cytotoxicity and blocking-serum activity to tumor antigen. Adv. Immunol. *18:* 209–277 (1974).

2   Baldwin, R. W.; Robbins, R. A.: Humoral factors abrogating cell-mediated immunity in the tumor-bearing host. Curr. Top. Microbiol. Immunol. *72:* 21–53 (1975).

3   Hellström, K. E.; Hellström, I.; Nepom, J. T.: Specific blocking factors – Are they important? Biochim. biophys. Acta *473:* 121–148 (1977).

4   Sjögren, H. O.; Hellström, I.; Bansal, S. C.; Hellström, K. E.: Suggestive evidence that the 'blocking antibodies' of tumor-bearing individuals may be antigen-antibody complexes. Proc. natn. Acad. Sci. USA *68:* 1372–1375 (1971).

5   Steele, G. Jr.; Ankerst, J.; Sjögren, H. O.: Alteration of in vitro antitumor activity of tumor-bearer sera by absorption with *Staphylococcus aureus,* Cowan I. Int. J. Cancer *14:* 83–92 (1974).

6   Steele, G. Jr.; Ankerst, J.; Sjögren, H. O.; Vang, J.; Lannerstad, O.: Absorption of blocking activity from human tumor-bearer sera by *Staphylococcus aureus,* Cowan I. Int. J. Cancer *15:* 180–189 (1975).

7   Bansal, S. C.; Bansal, B. R.; Rhoads, J. E. Jr.; Cooper, D. R.; Boland, J. P.; Mark, R.: Ex vivo removal of mammalian immunoglobulin G. Methods and immunological alterations. Int. J. artif. Organs *1:* 94–103 (1978).

8   Bansal, S. C.; Bansal, B. R.; Husberg, B.; Lindström, C.; Nylander, G.; Mark, R.; Sjögren, H. O.: Use of biological immunoabsorbents in the treatment of tumor host. Proc. Workshop on Therapeutic Plasma and Cytopheresis. Mayo Clinic/Mayo Foundation (in press, 1981).

9   Jones, F. R.; Yoshida, L. H.; Ladiges, W. C.; Kenny, M. A.: Treatment of feline leukemia and reversal of FeLV by ex vivo removal of IgG. Cancer *46:* 675–684 (1980).

10 Bansal, S. C.; Bansal, B. R.; Thomas, H. L.; Siegel, P. D.; Rhoads, J. E. Jr.; Cooper, D. R.; Terman, D. S.; Mark, R.: Ex vivo removal of serum IgG in a patient with colon carcinoma: Some biochemical, immunological, and histological observations. Cancer *42:* 1–18 (1978).

11 Sjögren, H. O.: Immunological aspects of colorectal cancer. Clin. Gastroenterol. *5:* 563–571 (1976).

12 Rosenberg, S. A. (ed.): Serologic Analysis of Human Cancer Antigens (Academic Press, New York 1980).

13 Bøyum, A.: Separation of leukocytes from blood and bone marrow. Scand. J. Clin. Lab. Invest. 21 (Suppl. 97): 31 (1968).

14 Malmström, P.; Jönsson, Å.; Hallberg, T.; Sjögren, H. O.: Counter-current distribution of lymphocytes from human peripheral blood in an aqueous two-phase system. I. Separation into subsets of lymphocytes bearing distinctive markers. Cell. Immunol. 53: 39–49 (1980).

15 Malmström, P.; Jönsson, Å.; Sjögren, A. O.: Counter-current distribution of lymphocytes from human peripheral blood in an aqueous two-phase system. II. Separation into subsets of lymphocytes with distinctive functions. Cell. Immunol. 53: 50–61 (1980).

16 Ey, P. L.; Prowse, S. J.; Jenkin, C. R.: Isolation of pure IgG 1, IgG 2a, and IgG 2b immunoglobulins from mouse serum using protein A-Sepharose. Immunochemistry 15: 429–436 (1978).

17 Albertsson, P.-Å.: Partition of cell particles and macromolecules (Wiley Interscience, New York 1971).

18 Lozzio, C. B.; Lozzio, B. B.: Human chronic myelogenous leukemia cell-line with positive Philadelphia chromosome. Blood 45: 321–334 (1975).

19 Andersson, L. C.; Nilsson, K.; Gamberg, C. G.: K 562 – A human erythroleukemic cell line. Int. J. Cancer 23: 143–147 (1979).

20 Bont, W. S.; De Vries, J. E.; Geel, M.; Van Dougen, A.; Loos, H. A.: Separation of human lymphocytes and monocytes by velocity sedimentation at unit gravity. J. immunol. Methods 29: 1–16 (1979).

Prof. Dr. H. O. Sjögren, The Wallenberg Laboratory, University of Lund, Box 7031, S-22007 Lund

Immunosuppressive Serum Factors

U. Kaboth

Medizin. Universitätsklinik, Abt. Hämatologie/Onkologie, Göttingen, FRG

Enhancement of the body's own tumor defense system is conceivable by means of immunostimulation or by elimination of an already impaired immune response to the tumor. In principle, both mechanisms can take place at the cellular level or along humoral paths – or through a coupled, humoral-cellular mechanism. Since a large body of evidence supports the existence of humoral factors that block the cellular immune response to the tumor, it seems appropriate, in the context of this symposium, to list all serum factors considered to be immunosuppressive and to concern ourselves somewhat more closely with the effects ascribed to them.

We must differentiate between specific and nonspecific factors (table I). The specific serum factors, which may have an immunosuppressive effect

Table I. Humoral serum factors with possible immunosuppressive effect in human neoplasias

1. *Specific*
   a) antibodies against tumor antigens
   b) circulating tumor antigens
   c) immune complexes formed by a) and b)

2. *Nonspecific*
   'Acute-phase proteins'
   (C-reactive protein, orosomucoid, haptoglobin, α-antitrypsin and others)
   Immunosuppressive α-globulins
   (IRA = immunoregulatory α-globulin, PAG = pregnancy-associated α-glycoprotein and others)
   Prostaglandins
   Interferon

3. Mediators liberated by immune reactions

4. ?

in tumor defense, include antibodies against tumor-specific antigens, the tumor-specific antigens themselves, and the immune complexes formed from them both. The nonspecific factors include the group of acute-phase proteins and the group of so-called immunosuppressive α-globulins which, in part, overlap. Further factors are possibly prostaglandins and interferon which, however, should perhaps be counted among the mediators that are released during cellular immune reactions.

Specific Factors

First, I will deal with the specific factors. *Hellström* and *Hellström* [28, 29] were able to show in vitro using a virus-induced mouse sarcoma (Moloney-sarcoma virus) that the cytotoxicity of the animal's lymphocytes for the tumor cells could be specifically blocked by adding the mouse serum. This observation could be reproduced by other authors, in particular *Baldwin, Bansal,* and *Sjörgren*, employing different tumor models, and also in in vitro investigations with serum and cells of human tumor bearers [4]. The blocking effect, which appears relatively early and simultaneously with the cytotoxic lymphocytes and increases with tumor spread, could be abolished by previous absorption of the inhibiting serum with the same type of tumor cells or by precipitating with anti-IgG [28, 49]. In addition, *Baldwin* and others observed in vivo an increase in tumor growth after administration of a hyperimmune serum against tumor-specific transplantation antigens [3, 4]. Thus, the mechanism was initially assumed to be a blocking action by an antibody directed against the tumor on the tumor cell itself. However, it had also been noticed that this blocking-serum effect disappears immediately or at least, for an antibody, very rapidly when the tumor is totally removed from an animal bearer; conversely, it does not disappear if some of the tumor is left. Because of this, the existence of additional factors was suspected. *Sjögren et al.* [49] and *Baldwin et al.* [2], were able to prove that the more important blocking effect clearly originates in the immune complexes. These can attack the target cells as well as the effector cells. The immune complex is fixed to the tumor cell by means of its antibody specificity or to the lymphocytes by the tumor-specific antigens they contain; in both cases they block a binding site (fig. 1). Finally, it was found, in particular by *Thompson et al.* [53], that freely circulating tumor antigens also inhibited the in vitro cytotoxicity of lymphocytes toward tumor cells, and that the reactivity of the lym-

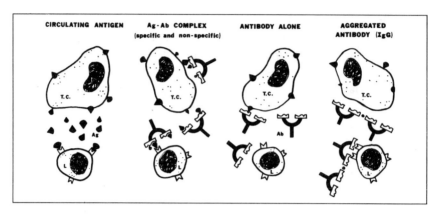

Fig. 1. Possible interaction mechanisms of tumor-specific antigen, antibody, and immune complexes with cellular tumor defense [4].

phocytes could be increased in vitro in patients with long-term tumors by repeated washing of the lymphocytes.

These and similar investigations by other researchers spoke for the existence of an additional blocking effect on the effector cells caused by free, circulating tumor antigens. The last-named mechanism most likely plays a role in advanced tumor stages with large tumor mass and a corresponding release of tumor-specific antigen. The course of the disease can be assumed to pass from a prevalence of antibodies to a predominance of circulating antigen (fig. 2).

Further, the phenomenon of the so-called "unblocking" must be mentioned. Using various experimental procedures, the blocking effect could be successfully abolished by administrating a presumedly immune serum from animals with tumors that had spontaneously regressed or the serum from animals that had been previously operated to remove the same type of tumor. This phenomenon (unblocking) is also described as specific. It is supposed that the excess antigen-binding sites on the immune complexes are occupied by factors in the unblocking serum. However, the mechanism is still unclarified and speculative. Finally, there is the possibility that the immune complexes, independent of their antigens, or that aggregated IgG molecules, bind the effector cells and thus exert a non-specific inhibitory effect (fig. 1).

Immune complexes are known to maximally precipitate at a certain concentration ratio of antigens to antibodies (equivalence point). In addition, the affinity of the antibody plays the role of a constant in the absolute

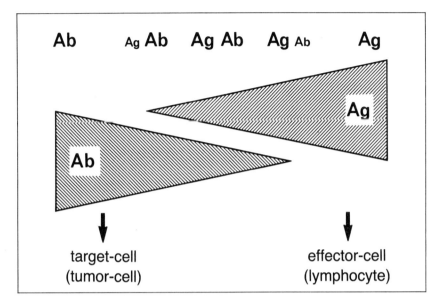

Fig. 2. Shifting balance of tumor-specific antibody, tumor-specific immune complex, and tumor-specific antigen in the course of tumor disease.

amount of precipitate. Soluble, circulating immune complexes, which can become effective humorally, appear especially in increasing, excess antigen. The composition of the immune complexes is very heterogeneous (table II). This causes methodologic problems, in particular the standardization of the many possible test procedures. The interpretation of the detected circulating immune complexes in individual cases is still problematic. Although immune complexes have been successfully correlated with the clinical course of many tumors and their prognoses, there are

Table II: Heterogeneity of circulating immune complexes

1. Molecular size, molecular weight, electric loading
2. Different antigens
3. Different antibody specificity, different immunoglobulin classes
4. Quantitative relation of antigen and antibody
   (antigen or antibody excess, equivalence zone)
5. Affinity of the antibody
6. Binding capacity for complement factors
7. Binding capacity for cell-membrane receptors

exceptions (see the paper of *Baldwin*). Since, as a rule, assignment to a definite and measurable tumor-specific antigen is not possible and because circulating immune complexes appear frequently in other illnesses, especially in infections, it is not yet possible to define with certainty whether the patient has more tumor-specific antigen or antibodies (fig. 2). When plasmapheresis is administered in the case of a certain tumor, the possibility must be considered that a temporary removal of immunosuppressive factors – or immune complexes – may indeed occur; but that subsequently the momentary equilibrium between tumor antigens and antibodies can shift in this or that direction, to the left or to the right, with desired or undesired consequences.

Nonspecific Factors

An immunosuppressive effect is also attributed to nonspecific factors in tumorous diseases. Having combed the literature, I have collated these factors in quite a long list (table III), without any claim to completeness or their true significance. It will only be possible to deal with a few of these factors in detail. Because of their large number, the different experimental procedures, and the many authors, it is more difficult to judge the immunosuppressive effect ascribed to nonspecific factors, and they are rarely confirmed by other investigators under comparable control tests. In my opinion, they are also generally less well-documented than specific factors.

The nonspecific factors [32, 54] include the acute-phase proteins and immunosuppressive α-globulins [1, 16, 17, 18] which overlap in part. It is well known that the acute-phase proteins and α-globulins are elevated in serum not only in cases of acute but also in cases of chronic inflammations and tumors. As so-called agglomerines, they are partially responsible for accelerating the blood sedimentation rate. The mechanism causing the increase of these proteins is unclear, as is the meaning of these changes, which supply the physician with a diagnostic parameter, however nonspecific it may be. It can be speculated that this is another feedback mechanism to regulate inflammable reactions, as is known, in the specific humoral system, for immunoglobulin synthesis.

The C-reactive protein derives its name from its ability to precipitate C-polysaccharide from pneumococci. It migrates in the gamma range, not in the alpha range; it can, with certainty, be delineated from the group of

Table III. Unspecific serum factors with possible immunosuppressive effects in human neoplasias

	References
C-reactive protein	Mortensen et al., 1975, 76, 77
Acid α_1-glycoprotein (Orosomocoid)	Chiur et al., 1977, Israel and Edelstein, 1978
Haptoglobin	Israel and Edelstein, 1978
(Transferrin)	Israel and Edelstein, 1978
α_2-Macroglobulin	Johannsen et al., 1974
Coeruloplasmin	Johannsen et al., 1974
Prealbumin	Johannsen et al., 1974
Fibrin-splitting products	Girmann et al., 1976, Edgington and Plow, 1976, Gramse et al., 1977
Fibrinogen	?
α_1-Antitrypsin	Arora et al., 1978, Bata et al., 1980
IRA (immunoregulatory α-globulins)	Cooperband et al., 1972, 76
NIP (normal immunosuppressive protein)	Nelken 1973
SAA (serum amyloid A protein)	Husby and Natvig, 1974, Benson et al., 1975
PAG (pregnancy-associated α_2-glycoprotein)	Schoultz et al. 1973, 74, Damber et al., 1975, Than et al., 1975, Stimson 1976, Bauer, Bohn, and Ax 1978
LDL-In (low-density lipoprotein inhibitor)	Curtis and Edgington, 1976
Lymphocyte-inhibition factor	Schumacher et al., 1974
RIF (rosette-inhibition-factor)	Chisari and Edgington, 1975, 76
SIF (serum-inhibition-factor)	Brattig and Berg, 1976, 78
Prostaglandin (E_2)	Smith et al. 1971, Gordon et al., 1976, Lomnitzer et al., 1976, Braun and Ishizuka 1971, Henney et al., 1972
Interferon	Lindahl-Magnusson et al., 1972, Brodeur and Merigan, 1975, Gisler et al. 1975, Chester et al., 1973, Johnson et al., 1975

immunosuppressive factors in the alpha range. Formerly it played, because of its nonspecificity, an unjustified role in the diagnosis of rheumatism (C-reactive protein, CRP). It binds selectively T-cells and suppresses the mixed lymphocyte reaction in the human system as well as the T-cell rosette formation [39, 40, 41]. Both effects can be canceled by adding C-polysaccharide. Orosomucoid (acidic α_1-glycoprotein) can arrest the mitogen- or alloantigen-induced lymphocyte proliferation [15]. A suppression of the lymphocytes' ability to be stimulated by PHA was found by *Israel* and *Edelstein* [32] for orosomucoid and haptoglobin, and, surprisingly, also for transferrin. Whereas the transferrin level is, as a rule, not elevated in inflammations and tumors, haptoglobin is always increased. Although one of the acute-phase proteins, haptoglobin's special function is the unbinding and removal of hemolysis hemoglobins. Further, the fibrinogen degradation products are also ascribed an immunosuppressive effect (suppression of the PHA stimulatability, the early lymphocyte activation, and leukocyte migration) [21, 23, 27]. Suppression of lymphocyte transformation was also observed in vitro for α_2-macroglobulin, coeruloplasmin, and prealbumin [33]. However, a number of serum proteins can unbind PHA and consequently disturb the PHA stimulation in vitro by themselves [38]. In particular we should refrain from including those, for which only the fact that they suppress PHA stimulation is known, among the potential immunosuppressive serum factors. In inflammations and tumors, α_1-antitrypsin is clearly elevated; it is a typical, acute-phase protein. α_1-Antitrypsin has been proven to have an immunosuppressive effect. It arrests antibody-plaque binding and the mitogen and allogen cell-induced transformation of lymphocytes [1a, 4a]. Proof for the immunosuppressive effect of fibrinogen was not found in the literature.

After the first discoveries in the 1960s on the use of an α_2 fraction to suppress transplant rejection in animal experiments, *Cooperband et al.* [16, 17, 18] found an immunosuppressive effect of a human α-globulin fraction at the cellular level (PHA stimulation of lymphocytes, mixed lymphocyte reaction, formation of MIF). They termed these serum factors IRA (immunoregulatory alphaglobulin). Subsequent partial purification of the IRA yielded numerous other fractions with different suppressive effects. However, no one single fraction could be successfully shown to be either singly or at least predominantly responsible for the proven immunosuppressive effect. Later, a dialyzable 0.6 S-polypeptide with immunosuppressive effect was successfully isolated, but this was associated with the α_1-, α_2-, and β-fractions [43]. The relationships between IRA, NIP (normal immunosuppressive protein), SAA (serum amyloid-A protein), and several other factors are unclear; overlapping or a combined immunosuppressive effect of partial fractions are possible.

In the group of nonspecific factors, the PAG (pregnancy-associated α_2-glycoprotein, see table IV), a protein that has been thoroughly characterized, is especially interesting. PAG is an α_2-globulin that is normally present in serum. But during pregnancy or medication with estrogen, PAG increases by a factor greater than 10, at times even reaching a factor of 60. An immunosuppressive effect has been ascribed to PAG, and supported by in vitro investigations particularly in connection with the absence of

Table IV. PAG (= pregnancy-associated α_2-glycoprotein)

Synonyms	References
Xm-factor	Berg and Bearn, 1966
Pa 1	MacLaren, 1966
Serum factor Xh	Bundschuh, 1966
Pregnancy protein 3	Bohn, 1971
Pregnancy-zone protein	Straube et al., 1972
PZ (pregnancy-zone protein)	von Schoultz and Stigbrand, 1973
Pregnancy-associated globulin	Horne et al., 1973
α_2-Pregnoglobulin	Berne, 1973
Pregnancy-associated α-macroglobulin	Stimsons and Sinclair, 1974

maternal rejection to the fetus. Many groups have been able to prove a suppression of the stimulatability of the T-cells in lymphocyte transformation tests [5, 20, 46, 51, 52]. Later *Bauer et al.* [5] showed a reduced formation of MSF (macrophage-slowing factor) in an electropheresis mobility test following pretreatment of the lymphocytes with PAG. Moreover, the presence of PAG on the lymphocyte membrane could be proven [5] by fluorescence optics. In many tumorous illnesses this protein is clearly elevated, although not to the same extent as during pregnancy, and it correlates well with the clinical course of the disease (for overview see [6, 8]).

Prostaglandin E_2 (overview in [25]) enhances local vasodilatation, vascular permeability and thus local edema [19], and in addition pain production through bradykinin and histamine [22]. On the other hand, it suppresses mitogen-induced lymphocyte proliferation [50], the formation of lymphokine [26, 36], direct cytolysis by activated T-lymphocytes [30], as well as the formation of antibodies [11], which can be measured by the Jerne-Plaque assay. It seems, therefore, surprising that only a few controlled investigations have been made to test the use of prostaglandin-suppressors in chemotherapy, at least as additional drugs.

Besides its well-known antiviral and general antiproliferative effect, interferon (see overview [9]) has been proven to have immunoregulatory features. For tumor defense, it is partially useful but also partially impairing (table V). Interferon *enhances* the expression of the histocompatability antigens, the cytotoxic activity of T-cells [35], the phagocytic ability of macrophages, and the activity of NK-cells [55]. Conversely, it *suppresses* the mitogen- and allogen-induced lymphocyte proliferation, the antibody formation in vivo and in vitro [12, 24, 34], which can also be measured by

Table V. Interferon

Acts
Antiviral
Antiproliferative
Immunomodulatory

Enhances
Expression of histocompatibility antigens
Cytotoxic activity of T-cells
Phagocytosis by macrophages
Activity of natural-killer cells

Inhibits
Mitogen- and allogen-induced lymphocyte proliferation
Antibody production in vivo
Antibody production in vitro
Jerne-Plaque formation (primary and secondary response)
Attack of natural-killer cells to T-cell membrane

---

the Jerne-Plaque formation (primary and secondary responses) as a parameter for a specific B-cell proliferation [13]. Interferon can protectively suppress the effect of the NK-cells on the target cell membrane [37], i.e., the stimulating effect on the NK-cells may be thereby canceled.

Similarly to RIF and SIF, prostaglandins and interferon can be considered, in the broader sense of the term, to be mediators released during the immune reactions. This will be treated in detail elsewhere. Possibly other immunoregulatory factors exist which have not yet been identified, but which can intercede so that tumor defense takes this or that direction (table I).

I have attempted to show that the basic concept of treating tumorous illnesses with plasmapheresis rests on numerous experimental facts of varying solidity. It is very difficult to evaluate the immunoregulatory effects of the individual factors on the basis of literature. In particular, it cannot be answered yet whether the immunosuppressive phenomena measured in vitro in human tumorous diseases are quantitatively so significant that the removal of certain serum factors is justified in tumor patients, or is, at least, of use in certain situations.

Nevertheless, the large body of evidence for the presence of immunosuppressive factors in tumorous illnesses encourages us to test these experimentally proven phenomena by the clinical application of plasmapheresis. As we have seen, this is now in progress.

References

1a Arora, P. K.; Miller, H. C.: α_1-Antitrypsin is an effector of immunological stasis. Nature *274:* 589–590 (1978).

1   Ashikawa, K.; Inoue, K.; Shimizu, T.; Ishibashi, Y.: An increase of serum alpha-globulin in tumor-bearing hosts and its immunological significance. Jap. J. exp. Med. *41:* 339–355 (1971).

2   Baldwin, R. W.; Price, M. R.; Robins, R. A.: Blocking of lymphocyte-mediated cytotoxicity for rat-hepatoma cells by specific antigen-antibody complexes. Nature new Biol. *238:* 185–187 (1972).

3   Baldwin, R. W.: Immunobiological aspects of chemical carcinogenesis. Adv. Cancer Res. *18:* 1–76 (1973).

4   Bansal, S. C.; Bansal, B. R.; Boland, J. P.: Blocking and Unblocking Serum Factors in Neoplasia. Current topics in microbiology and immunology pp. 45–76 (Springer-Verlag, Berlin, Heidelberg, New York 1976).

4a Bata, J.; Cordier, G.; Revillard, J.-P.; Bonneau, M.; Latour, M.: Modulation of lymphocyte responses by serum protease-antiprotease systems. In Touraine et al. (eds)., Transplantation and Clinical Immunology XI, pp. 59–70 (Excerpta Medica Amsterdam, Oxford, Princeton 1980).

5   Bauer, H. W.; Bohn, H.; Ax, W.: Immunologische Potenz des schwangerschaftsassoziierten Alpha$_2$-Glykoproteins (Alpha$_2$-PAG). Onkologie *1:* 119–123 (1978).

6   Bauer, H. W.: Das schwangerschaftsassoziierte α_2-Glykoprotein (α_2-PAG). Ein möglicher Marker zur Tumorverlaufskontrolle? Onkologie *4:* 183–186 (1980).

7   Benson, M. D.; Aldo-Benson, M. A.; Shirhama, T.; Borel, Y.; Cohen, A. S.: Suppression of in vitro antibody response by a serum factor (SAA) in experimentally induced amyloidosis. J. exp. Med. *142:* 236–241 (1975).

8   Bohn, H.; Bauer, H. W.: Schwangerschaftsassoziiertes α_2-Glykoprotein (α_2-PAG): Bedeutung seiner Bestimmung bei malignen Erkrankungen. Laboratoriumsblätter (Behring-Werke) *3:* 119–126 (1979).

9   Borden, E. C.: Interferons: Rationale for Clinical Trials in Neoplastic Disease. Ann. intern. Med. *91:* 472–479 (1979).

10 Brattig, N.; Berg, P. A.: Serum-inhibitory factors (SIF) in patients with acute and chronic hepatitis and their clinical significance. Clin. exp. Immunol. *25:* 40–49 (1976).

11 Braun, W.; Ishizuka, M.: Antibody formation: Reduced responses after administration of excessive amounts of nonspecific stimulators. Proc. natn. Acad. Sci. USA *68:* 114 (1971).

12 Brodeur, B. R.; Merigan, T. C.: Mechanism of the suppressive effect of interferon on antibody synthesis in vivo. J. Immun. *114:* 1323–1328 (1975).

13 Chester, T. J.; Paucker, K.; Merigan, T. C.: Suppression of mouse antibody producing spleen cells by various interferon preparations. Nature *246:* 92–94 (1973).

14 Chisari, F.V.; Edgington, T. S.: Lymphocyte E-rosette inhibitory factor: A regulatory serum lipoprotein. J. exp. Med. *142:* 1092–1107 (1975).

15 Chiu, K. M.; Mortensen, R. F.; Osmand, A. P.; Gewurz, H.: Interactions of alpha$_1$-acid glycoprotein with the immune system. I. Purification and effects upon lymphocyte responsiveness. Immunology *32:* 997–1005 (1977).

16 Cooperband, S. R.; Davis, R. C.; Schmid, K.; Mannick, J. A.: Competitive blockade of lymphocyte stimulation by a serum-immunoregulatory alpha-globulin (IRA). Transplant. Proc. *1:* 516–523 (1969).

17 Cooperband, S. R.; Badger, A. M.; Davis, R. C.; Schmid, K.; Mannick, J. A.: The effect of immunoregulatory α-globulin (IRA) upon lymphocytes in vitro. J. Immun. *109:* 154–163 (1972).

18   Cooperband, S. R.; Nimberg, R.; Schmid, K.; Mannick, J. A.: Humoral immunosup-
      pressive factors. Transplant. Proc. *8:* 225–242 (1976).
19   Crunkhorn, P.; Willis, A. L.: Actions and interactions of prostaglandin administered
      intradermally in rats and in man. Br. J. Pharmacol. *36:* 216 (1969).
20   Damber, M.-G.; Schoultz, B., von; Stigbrand, T.; Tärnvik, A.: Inhibition of the mixed
      lymphocyte reaction by the pregnancy-zone protein. FEBS Lett. *58:* 29–32 (1975).
21   Edgington, T. S.; Plow, E. F.: Suppression of lymphocyte function by physiological
      cleavage peptides of human fibrinogen (Abstract). Fed. Proc. *35:* 1318 (1976).
22   Ferreira, S. H.: Prostaglandins, aspirin-like drugs, and analgesia. Nature new Biol. *240:*
      200 (1972).
23   Girmann, G.; Pees, H.; Schwarze, G.; Scheurlen, P. G.: Immunosuppression by mi-
      cromolecular fibrinogen-degradation products in cancer. Nature, Lond. *259:* 399–401
      (1976).
24   Gisler, R. H.; Lindahl, P.; Gresser, I.: Effects of interferon on antibody synthesis in
      vitro. J. Immun. *113:* 438–444 (1974).
25   Goodwin, J. S.; Husby, G.; Williams, R. C., Jr.: Prostaglandin-E and Cancer Growth.
      Cancer Immunol. Immunother. *8:* 3–7 (1980).
26   Gordon, D.; Bray, M.; Morley, J.: Control of lymphocyte secretion by prostaglandins.
      Nature *262:* 461 (1976).
27   Gramse, M.; Löffler, C.; Schmidt, M.; Havemann, K.: Die Bildung niedermolekularer
      Fibrinogenopeptide durch granulozytäre Elastase und ihr Einfluß auf Lymphozyten-
      proliferation, Granulozyten- und Makrophagenmigration (Abstract). Z. Immun.
      Forsch. *153:* 302 (1977).
28   Hellström, I.; Hellström, K. E.: Studies on cellular immunity and its serum-mediated
      inhibition in Moloney virus-induced mouse sarcomas. Int. J. Cancer *4:* 587–600
      (1969).
29   Hellström, I.; Hellström, K. E.: Colony-inhibition studies on blocking and non-block-
      ing serum effects on cellular immunity to Moloney sarcomas. Int. J. Cancer *5:* 195–201
      (1970).
30   Henney, C. C.; Bourne, H. R.; Lichtenstein, L. M.: The role of cyclic 3' 5'-adenosine
      monophosphate in the specific cytolytic activity of lymphocytes. J. Immun. *108:* 1526
      (1972).
31   Husby, G.; Natvig, J. B.: A serum component related to non-immunoglobulin amyloid
      protein-AS, a possible precursor of the fibrils. J. clin. Invest. *53:* 1054–1061 (1974).
32   Israel, L.; Edelstein, R.: In vivo and in vitro studies on nonspecific blocking factors of
      host origin in cancer patients. Israel J. med. Scis. *14:* 105–130 (1978).
33   Johannsen, R.; Haupt, H.; Bohn, H.; Heide, K.; Seiler, F. R.; Schwick, H. G.: Inhibi-
      tion of the mixed leukocyte culture (MLC) by proteins: Mechanism and specificity of
      the reaction. Z. Immun. Forsch. *152:* 280–285 (1976).
34   Johnson, H. M.; Smith, B. G.; Baron, S.: Inhibition of the primary in vitro antibody
      response by interferon preparations. J. Immun. *114:* 403–409 (1975).
35   Lindahl, P.; Leary, P.; Gresser, I.: Enhancement by interferon of the specific cytotoxic-
      ity of sensitized lymphocytes. Proc. natn. Acad. Sci. USA *69:* 721–725 (1972).
36   Lomnitzer, R.; Rabson, A. R.; Koornhof, H. J.: The effects of cyclic-AMP on leuko-
      cyte-inhibitory factor (LIF) production and on the inhibition of leukocyte migration.
      Clin. exp. Immunol. *24:* 42–48 (1976).
37   Moore, M.; White, W. J.; Potter, M. R.: Modulation of target-cell susceptibility to
      human natural-killer cells by interferon. Int. J. Cancer *25:* 565–572 (1980).
38   Morse, J. H.: Immunological studies of phytohaemagglutinin. I. Reaction between
      phytohaemagglutinin and normal sera. Immunology *14:* 713–724 (1968).
39   Mortensen, R. F.; Osmand, A. P.; Gewurz, H.: Effects of C-reactive protein on the

lymphoid system. I. Binding to thymus-dependent lymphocytes and alteration of their functions. J. exp. Med. *141:* 821–839 (1975).

40   Mortensen, R. F.; Gewurz, H.: Effects of C-reactive protein on the lymphoid system. II. Inhibition of mixed lymphocyte reactivity and generation of cytotoxic lymphocytes. J. Immun. *116:* 1344–1350 (1976).

41   Mortensen, R. F.; Braun, D.; Gewurz, H.: Effects of C-reactive protein on lymphocyte functions. III. Inhibition of antigen-induced lymphocyte stimulation and lymphokine production. Cell. Immunol. *28:* 59–68 (1977).

42   Nelken, D.: Normal immunosuppressive protein (NIP). J. Immun. *110:* 1161–1162 (1973).

43   Occhino, J. C.; Glasgow, A. H.; Cooperband, S. R.; Mannick, J. A.: Isolation of an immunosuppressive peptide fraction from human plasma. J. Immun. *110:* 685–694 (1973).

44   Oppenheim, J. J.; Rosenstreich, D. L.: Signals Regulating in Vitro Activation of Lymphocytes. Prog. Allergy, *20:* 65–194 (1976).

45   Rogers, T. J.; Nowowiejski, I.; Webb, D. R.: Partial Characterization of a Prostaglandin-Induced Suppressor Factor. Cell. Immunology *50:* 82–93 (1980).

46   Schoultz, B., von; Stigbrand, T.; Tärnvik, A.: Inhibition of PHA-induced lymphocyte stimulation by the pregnancy-zone protein. FEBS Lett. *38:* 23–26 (1973).

47   Schoultz, B., von; Stigbrand, T.: Purification of the 'Pregnancy Zone' protein. Acta obstet. gynec. scand. *52:* 51–57 (1973).

48   Schumacher, K.; Maerker-Alzer, G.; Wehmer, U.: A lymphocyte-inhibiting factor isolated from normal human liver. Nature, Lond. *251:* 655–656 (1974).

49   Sjögren, H. O.; Hellström, I.; Bansal, S. C.; Hellström, K. E.: Suggestive evidence that 'blocking antibodies' of tumor-bearing individuals may be antigen-antibody complexes. Proc. natn. Acad. Sci. USA *68:* 1372–1375 (1971).

50   Smith, J. W.; Steiner, A. L.; Parker, C. W.: Human lymphocyte metabolism: Effects of cyclic and non-cyclic nucleotides on stimulation by phytohemagglutinin. J. clin. Invest. *50:* 442 (1971).

51   Stimson, W. H.: Studies on the immunosuppressive properties of a pregnancy-associated α-macroglobulin. Clin. exp. Immunol. *25:* 199–206 (1976).

52   Than, G. N.; Csaba, I. F.; Szabo, D. G.; Paal, M.; Ambrus, M.; Bajtai, G.: In vitro suppression effect of pregnancy-associated α_2-glycoprotein on the lymphocyte blastogenic response. IRCS med. Sci. *3:* 309 (1975).

53   Thompson, D. M. P.; Steele, K.; Alexander, P.: The presence of tumor-specific membrane antigens in the serum of rats with chemically induced sarcomata. Brit. J. Cancer *27:* 27–34 (1973).

54   Tomasi, T. B.: Serum factors which suppress the immune response. In Lucas (ed.), Regulatory mechanisms in lymphocyte activiation; Leucocyte culture conference, Arizona Medical Center, pp. 219–248 (New York 1977).

55   Zarling, J. M.; Eskra, L.; Borden, E. C.; Horoszewicz, J.; Carter, W. A.: Activation of human natural-killer cells cytotoxic for human leukemia cells by purified interferon. J. Immun. *123:* 63–70 (1979).

Prof. Dr. U. Kaboth, Medizin. Universitätsklinik, Abt. Hämatologie/Onkologie, Robert-Koch-Str. 40, D-3400 Göttingen

III. Tumor Immune Diagnosis

Chairmen:
K. Hoeffken, Essen and *J.-H. Beyer*, Göttingen

Humoral Immunodiagnosis in Carcinoma Patients

U. E. Nydegger and P. J. Spaeth

Zentrallaboratorium, Blutspendedienst, SRK, Bern, Schweiz

Normally the growth of malignant cells in a host organism is controlled by regulating cellular and humoral mechanisms. Macrophages and a specialized subpopulation of lymphocytes, the cytotoxic killer cells, are assumed to be able to directly stop tumor growth; however, their function can, in turn, be arrested by blocking factors, e.g., antibodies and/or immune complexes [1, 2].

Human malignant cells have been shown to possess antigen determinants that can produce a specific immune response. Such tumor-specific antigens could combine with antibodies on the cell surface or while circulating in the blood plasma and form immune complexes.

A considerable number of human tumors, above all breast cancer, cancer of the colon, as well as certain melanomas, lymphomas, and forms of leukemia, are often associated with circulating immune complexes (CIC).

In certain cases the blood concentration of such complexes also corresponds to the clinical degree of tumor proliferation, and a quantitation of CIC could be used for prognostic purposes. The fact that therapeutic removal of such complexes has led to the reduction of the tumor mass in certain patients [3, 4] further indicates their importance in tumor growth. Furthermore, tumor growth is occasionally accompanied by an equilibrium disturbance of the complement system, as has been confirmed in patients with Hodgkin's disease and leukemia.

This paper concerns itself with the role that a registration of all the dependent factors cited above could play in tumor diagnostics. Following this we deal with the detection of the most important tumor antigens and the reaction of the host to these antigens.

Cellular Tumor Diagnostics

To register the cellular interactions [5] the following tests can be considered:

(a) Cellular immune response to a tumor can be documented by injecting tumor extracts intracutaneously. This test involves a skin reaction of the late type with maximal reddening and induration for approximately 24–48 h after the injection. These reactions, however, are non-constant, frequently remain very discrete, and thus are difficult to interpret. Moreover, such tests are potentially dangerous, since, under certain conditions, tumor viruses could be transfered. For these reasons, test systems have become accepted in recent years which make registration possible of the lymphocytic immune response to tumor cells in vitro.

(b) Measurement of the cytotoxic capacity of the patient's lymphocytes as opposed to that of his tumor cells or tumor cells of similar histologic origin.

(c) Measurement of tumor cell-induced lymphoblasts from the patient's lymphocytes.

(d) Evaluation of lymphokines, mediator substances secreted by lymphocytes, whose production is stimulated by the tumor cells.

The results of these tests are positive in numerous cases, thus demonstrating that a patient, as a rule, is capable of producing an immunologic reaction to his own tumor cells, although it may be weak or often not very specific.

However, it must be noted that there is still no proof available of the tumoricidal usefulness of a cellular immune reaction. Nor have any of these tests reached the stage of general validity required by the clinician for diagnostic methods.

Humoral Diagnosis of Tumors

We must differentiate between detection of substances released by tumor cells and detection of pathologic deviations in the humoral immune response to the tumor.

Tumor Cell Products

Among those substances originating in the tumor, the monoclonal myeloma proteins and the corresponding Bence-Jones proteins are characteristic for multiple myeloma. Numerous enzymes, isoenzymes, hormones, and also catecholamines have assumed an important role in tumor diagnostics, especially when it is a question of ectopic localization of the tumor.

Most of the quantitative detections of tumor antigens are now made with the aid of a special radioimmunologic technique. These are, however, by no means restricted to the immunology laboratory [6]. Although such substances are detected with heterologous antibodies, they are generally not termed tumor-specific antigens. Opposed to these are the substances that are labeled tumor-associated antigens. The two most important of these and still the only ones actually usable for diagnostic purposes are the α_1-fetoprotein and the carcinoembryonic antigen (CEA). Both are oncofetal, i.e., abundantly present in the fetus and normally only in a weak concentration in the adult; this concentration, however, again greatly increases in case of a malignant transformation of a tumor. An attractive thesis explains this by genetic repression at birth and a depression that proceeds with a cellular dedifferentiation. Here it should be mentioned that α_1-fetoproteins and CEA are not antigens in the strict sense of the term, for there is no proof of an immune reaction in a homologous system.

α_1-Fetoprotein is primarily useful for diagnosing hepatoma. Malignant teratomas require differential diagnosis, since the values for α_1-fetoprotein do not drastically increase as a rule.

In 1965 *Gold* and *Freedman* isolated the carcinoembryonic antigen (CEA) from an adenocarcinoma in the large intestine. The CEA-plasma concentration was measured by radioimmunoassay with a sensitivity of 1–2 ng/ml.

In the early 70s the detection of CEA was closely tied to the hope for a reliable test for diagnosing cancer patients. Nowadays the test is preferentially used to register tumor masses that are already sizable, e.g., metastases of the breast or lung carcinoma. The CEA test [7] may also be useful to evaluate the success of a surgical resection of a tumor or chemotherapy. In such a manner, 303 patients with histologically positive adenocarcinoma of the gastro-intestinal tract were monitored postoperatively by analyzing the changes in CEA-serum concentrations over time. Early prognosis of a recurrence or metastases was made possible by the course

Table I. Serologic diagnosis with important human cancer antigens [after 5 and 6]

Antigen	Frequent test system	Value
CEA[1]	RIA[2]	Prognosis of recurrence
α_1-Fetoprotein	Immunoprecipitation	Diagnosis of hepatoma
Brain-tumor antigen	Cytotoxicity	Diagnostic
Sarcoma antigen	Cytotoxicity	Experimental
Lung-tumor antigen	RIA	Experimental
Leukemia antigen	Supravital staining fluorescence-activated cell-sorter	Experimental
Melanoma antigen	Complement fixation RIA	Experimental

[1] Carcinoembryonic antigen
[2] Radioimmunoassay

tendencies revealed by the curve monitoring CEA levels. Prognoses of recurrence based on renewed elevation of the CEA concentration were made up to 10 months in advance of a clinical diagnosis. These findings were confirmed by a second-look operation or other diagnostic methods. Further, the tendencies of the CEA course permitted differentiation between a generalized formation of metastases and local recurrence or a limited metastasis in the area of the local recurrence [8].

Other important tumor antigens are listed in table I.

Recently an attempt was made to utilize the appearance of CEA on tumor cells to determine the localization of the tumor. In this connection, *Mach et al.* [9] injected radioactively labeled anti-CEA antibodies into 27 carcinoma patients. The patients were then tested for tissue-bound radioactivity by means of a scintillation camera: in 11 patients tumor-bound radioactivity could be localized 48 h after the injection. This method is still in the experimental stage.

Tumor-Induced Humoral Immunity

Although the origin of tumor-specific antigens on the surface of the tumor cell is still controversial, it nevertheless seems likely that the cancerous organism defends itself by forming specific antibodies against these antigens. For the present, it can be assumed that such a formation of antibodies should have a tumoricidal effect. Under certain circumstances, however, such defense mechanisms could also be harmful to the host organism. One example of this is the fact that antibodies can mask the antigen by reacting with it, making the tumor cells unidentifiable to the other defense mechanisms. Furthermore, antibodies could react with the antigens released by the tumor cells and form CIC. Such complexes containing tumor antigens and antibodies can then precipitate in the tissue or bind the lymphocyte receptors, and thus impair the function of the structure involved.

As is the case in chronic virus infections or autoimmune diseases, antigens are chronically released in malignant diseases. The persistent antigenemia, combined with continual production of antibodies, lead to continuous formation of immune complexes. As yet there is no conclusive proof that such mechanisms exist. There are reasons to believe that tumor antigens appear as components of certain antigen-antibody complexes in carcinoma patients [10, 11].

Detection of Circulating Immune Complexes

There is nowadays a plethora of methods for detecting CIC (overview in [12]). Individual immunology laboratories have specialized in this or that test. Thus, the informed lab director often has to rely on anecdotal reports when choosing the best method for his own laboratory. Criteria such as specificity, sensitivity, and reproducibility have to be weighed against technical and time costs. In individual cases it can be a question of whether two or three tests can be carried out simultaneously on a patient's serum or sample, since not all tests can detect exactly the same type of immune complexes; in other words, if the sera of a patient population are examined for CIC with different methods, different percentage values will often be given for positive tests. The two methods used most frequently in carcinoma patients to detect presence of immune complexes are currently the C_{1q}-binding assay and the Raji-cell test.

Together with C_{1r} and C_{1s}, C_{1q} is the first component of complement. A globulin with molecular weight of 400,000 enters into a specific close combination with the immunoglobulins contained in the immune complexes. Figure 1 explains the principle of the C_{1q}-binding assay [13, 14] in more detail. Two test steps can be differentiated: first the test serum is mixed with EDTA for 30 min at 37° C; this produces a dissociation of the serum-C_{1qrs} complexes. The addition of EDTA in the C_{1q}-binding assay

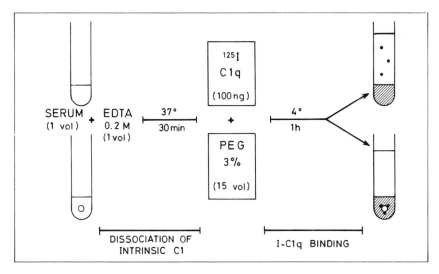

Fig. 1. The C_{1q} binding assay. Serum, containing immune complexes (left test tube below with o) or without immune complexes (test tube above left), is mixed with EDTA to break up the serum's own C_{1qrs} complex. Subsequently radioactively labeled C_{1q} and polyethylene glycol (PEG) is added, incubated, and centrifuged. Immune complexes bind C_{1q} (right, below), whereas normal serum does not, and C_{1q} is removed with the supernatant.

hinders inclusion of radioactively labeled C_{1q} in the serum's own C_{1qrs} complex. In a second step the radioactively labeled (^{125}I) C_{1q} and polyethylene glycol (PEG, final concentration of 2.5%) are added, and the mixture is incubated further for 1 h at 4° C. Under these conditions free ^{125}I-C_{1q} remains in solution, whereas ^{125}I-C_{1q}, that is fixed to macromolecular immune complexes, precipitates.

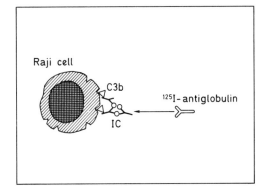

Fig. 2. The Raji cell test. The third complement component, designated by the small triangle, forms the bridge between C3b receptors on the Raji cells and the immune complexes. After the Raji cells are incubated with serum containing immune complexes, the cells are washed and in a second phase incubated with radioactively labeled antiglobulin antibodies. The latter can only bind those cells that have previously fixed immune complexes (positive test).

The most successful cellular test is the Raji-cell test [15] (fig. 2). This is a radioimmune test which is based on the binding of cellular complement receptors with immune complexes containing complement. Raji cells have surface receptors for the Fc fragment of immunoglobulins as well as for C3 and C3b. The test serum is incubated with the cells; these are then washed and incubated with radioactively labeled anti-human immunoglobulin antiserum. The absorbance of radioactive material on the cell surface provides a way of measuring the amount of complexed immunoglobulin bound on the cell surface.

These two methods for detecting immune complexes as well as 16 other tests were recently tested more closely in an international comparative study carried out under the auspices of *WHO* [16]. Special emphasis was placed on the question of how comparable test results are derived by different methods. In some laboratories the test results are expressed as percentages of the norm. Often the values found in normal control groups, which are always lower, are subtracted from patient results, or else calculated as a factor of Farr's formula.

$$\text{Farr's formula: } \% \text{ binding} = 100 - \frac{(100 - \% \text{ of sample}) \times 100}{100 - \% \text{ of control}}$$

The comparability of the methods has recently been improved even further. For example, if native immunoglobulin is heated for 20 min at $60°$ C, polymers are formed which, in most of their properties, are very similar to an antigen-antibody complex. Standard curves can be set up for the Raji-cell test and the C_{1q}-binding assay, which permit their results to be expressed as mg/ml of detected AHG (aggregated human gamma-globulin).

In such a manner *Day et al.* [17] found different amounts of immune complexes in different forms of cancer (table II). Recently a study group was formed under *WHO* auspices with the aim of producing an international reference standard and the Central Laboratory of the Swiss Red Cross was commissioned by this group to distribute two different standards: AHG and tetanus toxoid – antitetanus toxoid complexes.

The C_{1q}-binding assay has become a widely accepted method of detecting immune complexes in cancer patients [18]. In a larger study in 495 patients, abnormally high immune complex values were found in 128 patients with melanoma, in 41 with lung cancer, in 37 with cancer of the colon, and in 91 with breast cancer; similarly, a retrospective study in 22 breast cancer patients showed higher C_{1q}-binding activity values in most of

Table II. A selection of published cases of cancer patients with circulating immune complexes

Type of tumor	No. cases	Reference no.
Melanoma	128	17
Breast cancer	91 + 22	17 + 20
Gynecologic carcinomas	48	17
Colorectal carcinomas	37	17
Leukemia	97	21
Lymphomas	31	30
Hodgkin's lymphoma	23	22

the serum samples before mastectomy than was found postoperatively [19, 20].

Immune complexes are also observed in leukemia patients, as was clearly shown in a study of 467 serum samples from 230 leukemia patients [21]. Elevated C_{1q}-binding values were present in 40% of the patients with acute myeloid leukemia, in 23% of those with acute lymphatic leukemia, and in 46% of cases with acute predominance of myeloblasts during chronic myeloid leukemia. Conversely, just slightly over 10% patients, 12% in cases of chronic lymphatic and 13% in chronic myeloid leukemia, seemed to indicate presence of CIC. The C_{1q}-binding activity appears useful in the prognosis of remission. For example, in ¾ of the cases, without any detectable immune complexes, there was prompt remission of the disease, whereas only ½ of those cases with immune complexes entered into remission. Furthermore, monitoring of the course of disease in one and the same patient over several months showed that higher immune complexes were often observed when there was an abundance of myeloblasts, whereas the remission phases were associated with normal or only slightly elevated values (fig. 3).

Recently the serum and plasma samples of 6 patients with Hodgkin's disease were tested with four different methods for detecting immune complexes [22]. A positive and abnormal result from one or several of the applied tests was found in 90% of the symptomatically ill patients, in comparison with only 30% in the asymptomatic patients who were in the remission phase.

These clinical observations seem to be confirmed by animal experiments. It is possible to induce tumors that are invasive to different degrees in rats by injecting different amounts of sarcoma cells subcutaneously. If many cells are injected, tumors arise which quickly take a fatal course; if

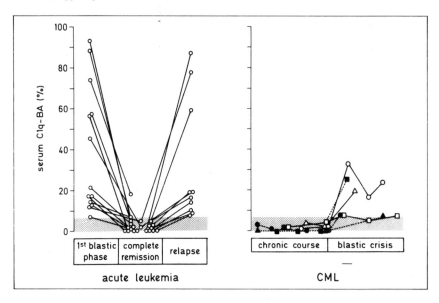

Fig. 3. Circulating immune complexes, detected by their C_{1q}-binding activity in acute and chronic myeloid leukemia. Quantities of myeloblasts and recurrences are more frequently associated with high C_{1q}-binding activity than is remission (with permission of [21]).

fewer cells are injected, tumors arise which, after reaching a maximal size, heal again. If during the evolution of such rat sarcomas, the animal sera are examined for immune complexes, a correlation is again found between tumor invasion and the quantity of circulating immune complexes (fig. 4). However, in cases with massive tumor invasion, the amount of immune complexes declined again [23].

Detection of the Activation of Complement

The complement system is a group of approximately 20 plasma proteins that react with each other in a coordinated way, similar to the coagulation system, so as to assume important effector tasks in the process of inflammation. The cytotoxic capacity of complement should also be mentioned in connection with certain problems in oncology [24]. For newer overviews about complement see references [25, 26, 27, 27a].

Immune complex and complement often react with each other. This can be a disadvantage for the host organism when the complement activa-

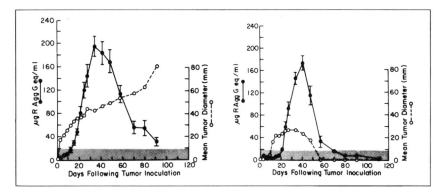

Fig. 4. Circulating immune complexes (•— — — —•) in the sarcoma-bearing rat. In the upper section of the figure the animals die from a steadily growing tumor (o— — — —o), whereas the animals in the lower section bear tumors only temporarily. In both cases the circulating immune complexes are observed approximately 6 weeks after inoculation of sarcoma cells (cited with the friendly permission of [23]).

tion leads to the formation of anaphylatoxin or other derivatives promoting inflammation. Conversely, it can also be advantageous in that the complement can change the size of the immune complexes [28] and thus favor its elimination.

Despite the great importance of this interaction between immune complex and complement, the study of the components of complement in cancer patients has only begun to spread within the last few years. One study found complement activation in 30% of the lymphoma patients [29], and abnormal concentration deviations of the 5th, 8th, and 9th components in 42 patients with acute leukemia, Hodgkin's disease, and sarcoma [31]. Furthermore, patients with lymphosarcoma and adenocarcinoma of the rectum had a C1-inhibitor deficit [32]. It was even proposed that the dosage of this control protein of complement could become important for diagnosis of recurrence.

Conclusions on the Significance of Plasma Exchange

The detection of certain cancer antigens as well as immune complexes and complement components have assumed a certain importance in recent times for the diagnosis of cancer.

Although series investigations have often found statistically significant correlations between the concentration of tumor antigens and CIC on the one hand, and the clinical extent of the disease on the other, high CEA or immune complex levels do not automatically prove presence of tumor in the individual patient. In addition, we are far from judging the presence of immune complexes as simply bad, and from this draw the conclusion that such complexes should be eliminated by means of plasma exchange of as large a volume as possible. The removal of large amounts of blood plasma in cases of elevated immune complexes will naturally also lead to a shift in the antigen-antibody ratio, since it is scarcely possible that equal amounts of free antigens and free antibodies will be removed during plasma exchange. Consequently in the case of re-formation of immune complexes, these could differ physicochemically and pathogenetically from those complexes present before plasma exchange. The effect of the chosen substitute fluid on the organism, which is usually fresh-frozen plasma, albumin, or a mixture of albumin and immunoglobulin, has barely been investigated.

Especially in cases where the removed plasma is substituted with plasma from a healthy donor, we must also consider the effect of additional complement components, which will then influence the re-formation of immune complexes.

Acknowledgment

The authors would like to express their sincere thanks to *Mrs. G. Balmer* for her very competent secretarial work.

References

1   Hellström, I.; Sjögren, H. O.; Warner, G.; Hellström, K. E.: Blocking of cell-mediated tumor immunity by sera from patients with growing neoplasms. Int. J. Cancer 7: 226 (1971).

2   Hellström, K. E.; Hellström, I.: Lymphocyte-mediated cytotoxicity and blocking serum activity to tumor antigens. Adv. Immunol. 18: 249 (1974).

3   Bansal, S. C., and Bansal, B. R.: Serum-blocking factors in tumor host. Are they important? Contr. Oncol., vol. 10, pp. 91–101 (Karger, Basel 1982).

4   Ray, P. K.; Clarke, L.; McLaughlin, D.; Allen, P.; Idiculla, A.; Mark, R.; Rhoads, J. E. Jr.; Basset, J. G.; Cooper, D. R.: Immunotherapy of cancer: Extracorporeal adsorption of plasma-blocking factors using nonviable Staphylococcus aureus Cowan I. Contr. Oncol., vol. 10, pp. 102–113 (Karger, Basel 1982).

5   Herberman, R. B.; McIntire, K. R.: Immunodiagnosis of cancer (Marcel Dekker, Inc., New York 1979).

6   Rosenberg, S. A. (ed.): Serologic analysis of human cancer antigens (Academic Press, Inc., London 1980).

7 CEA 'Roche' Test: In vitro-Test zur Prognose und Diagnosehilfe bei Karzinomen (Hoffmann-La Roche, Basel 1978).

8 Staab, H. J.; Anderer, F. A.; Stumpf, E.; Fischer, D.: Carcinoembryonales Antigen (CEA). Dt. med. Wschr. *102:* 1082 (1977).

9 Mach, J. P.; Carrel, S.; Forni, M.; Ritschard, J.; Donath, A.; Alberto, P.: Tumor localization of radiolabeled antibodies against carcinoembryonic antigen in patients with carcinoma. New Engl. J. Med. *303:* 5 (1980).

10 Baldwin, R. W.; Bowen, J. G.; Price, M. R.: Detection of circulating hepatoma D23 antigen and immune complexes in tumor-bearer serum. Brit. J. Cancer *28:* 16 (1973).

11 Kapsopoulou-Dominos, K.; Anderer, F. A.: Circulating carcinoembryonic antigen immune complexes in sera of patients with carcinomata of the gastro-intestinal tract. Clin. exp. Immunol. *35:* 190 (1979).

12 Nydegger, U. E.: Biological properties and detection of immune complexes in animal and human pathology. Rev. Physiol. Biochem. Pharmacol. *85:* 63 (1979).

13 Nydegger, U. E.; Lambert, P. H.; Gerber, H.; Miescher, P. A.: Circulating immune complexes in the serum in systemic lupus erythematosis and in carriers of hepatitis B antigen. J. clin. Invest. *54:* 297 (1974).

14 Zubler, R. H.; Lange, G.; Lambert, P. H.; Miescher, P. A.: Detection of immune complexes in unheated sera by a modified $125I$-C_{1q}-binding test. J. Immunol. *116:* 232 (1976).

15 Theophilopoulos, A. N.; Dixon, F. J.: The biology and detection of immune complexes. Adv. Immunol. *28:* 89 (1980).

16 Lambert, P. H. et al. (19 authors): A WHO collaborative study for the evaluation of eighteen methods for detecting circulating immune complexes in serum. J. clin. Lab. Immunol. *1:* 1 (1978).

17 Day, N. K.; Brandeis, W. E.: Relevance of circulating immune complexes in cancer sera. In: Peeters (ed.), Protides of biological fluids, p. 325 (Pergamon Press, Oxford 1979).

18 Baldwin, R. W.; Byers, V. S.; Robins, R. A.: Circulating immune complexes in cancer: Characterization and potential as tumour markers. Behring Inst. Mitt. *64:* 63ᵛ (1979).

19 Teshima, H.; Wanebo, H.; Pinsky, C.; Day, N. K.: Circulating immune complexes detected by $125I$-C_{1q}-deviation test in sera of cancer patients. J. clin. Invest. *59:* 1134 (1977).

20 Hoffken, K.; Meredith, I. D.; Robins, R. A.; Baldwin, R. W.; Davies, C. J.; Blamey, R. W.: Circulating immune complexes in patients with breast cancer. Br. med. J. *ii:* 218 (1977).

21 Carpentier, N.; Lange, G. T.; Fiere, D. M.; Fournie, G. I.; Lambert, P. H.; Miescher, P. A.: Clinical relevance of circulating immune complexes in human leukemia. Association in acute leukemia of the presence of immune complexes with unfavorable prognosis. J. clin. Invest. *60:* 874 (1977).

22 Amlot, P. L.; Pussell, B.; Slaney, J. M.; Williams, B. D.: Correlation between immune complexes and prognostic factors in Hodgkin's disease. Clin. exp. Immunol. *31:* 166 (1978).

23 Jennette, J. C.: Consistent fluctuations in quantitites of circulating immune complexes during progressive and regressive phases of tumor growth. Am. J. Path. *100:* 403 (1980).

24 Shearer, W. T.; Parker, C. W.: Antibody and complement modulation of tumor cell growth in vitro and in vivo. Fed. Proc. *37:* 2385 (1978).

25 Bitter-Suermann, D.: Zur Physiologie, Pathophysiologie und Klinik des Komplementsystems. SM *2:* 43 (1980).

26 Götze, O.; Mueller-Eberhard, H. J.: The alternative pathway of complement activation. Adv. Immunol. *24:* 1 (1976).

27   Fearon, D. T.; Austen, F. J.: Current concepts in immunology: The alternative pathway
      of complement – a system for host resistance to microbial infection. New Engl. J. Med.
      303: 259 (1980).
27a   Kazatchkine, M. O.; Nydegger, U. E.: The human alternative complement pathway:
      Biology and immunopathology of activation and regulation. Prog. Allergy (in press).
28   Czop, J.; Nussenzweig, V.: Studies on the mechanism of solubilization of immune
      precipitates by serum. J. exp. Med. *143:* 615 (1976).
29   Heier, H. E.; Carpentier, N. A.; Lambert, P. H.; Godal, T.: Quantitation of serum
      complement components and plasma C3d in patients with malignant lymphoma: Rela-
      tion to the stage of the tumor and circulating immune complexes. Int. J. Cancer *21:* 695
      (1978).
30   Heier, H. E.; Carpentier, N.; Lange, G.; Godal, T.: Circulating immune complexes in
      patients with malignant lymphomas and solid tumors. Int. J. Cancer *20:* 887 (1977).
31   Lichtenfeld, J. L.; Wiernick, P. H.; Mardiney, M. R.; Zarco, R. M.: Abnormalities of
      complement and its components in patients with acute leukemia, Hodgkin's disease,
      and sarcoma. Cancer Res. *36:* 3678 (1976).
32   Wintzer, G.; Koch, O.; Uhlenbruck, G.: Die Bedeutung von C1 Inactivator, alpha$_1$-
      Antichymotrypsin und Inter alpha-Trypsin Inhibitor in der Diagnostik und Nachsorge
      maligner Tumoren. Lab. Med. *4:* 134 (1980).

Dr. U. E. Nydegger, PD, Zentrallaboratorium, Blutspendedienst, SRK, Wankdorfstr. 10,
CH-3000 Bern 22

Immunological Procedures for Diagnosis and Monitoring the Course of Patients with Cancer

K. Havemann

Abteilung Hämatologie/Onkologie, Zentrum für Innere Medizin der Universität Marburg, FRG

The detection of tumor-associated antigens is of increasing importance for diagnosis and evaluating the course of patients with malignant tumors. The identification of tumor-associated antigens is almost entirely carried out by immunological methods with heterologous antisera. Depending on the concentration of the antigen in the tumor or serum, either rather insensitive immunoprecipitation methods or highly sensitive enzyme and radioimmune assays are applied. Numerous proteins are elevated in the serum of patients with cancer, which are clearly in excess of their concentration in healthy volunteers. However, in general, these tumor-associated antigens are neither neoantigens nor antigens, which are specific for a certain histological tumortype [3]. The list of these substances, also termed tumor markers, is long and can be expanded easily (table I).

Virus-associated antigens, oncofetal antigens, hormones, enzymes, metalbinding proteins, but also acute-phase proteins and coagulation factors have been described as tumor-associated antigens. With the possible exception of a few, these proteins are not identical with tumor-specific antigens. Beside the tumor-associated antigens, patients with tumors also show circulating immune complexes in their plasma. These complexes are composed of antibodies, complement components, and antigens, which so far have been characterized in only a few instances. Since the formation of antibody against these antigens implies a loss of tolerance, the antigens may represent true neoantigens.

Table I. Tumor-associated antigens in human malignancies

Virus-associated antigens	
Epstein-Barr-virus antigens	Burkitts lymphoma
	Nasopharyngeal carcinoma
Herpes-simplex-virus antigens	Carcinoma of the cervix
	HNO tumors
Mouse mamma-tumor-virus antigens	Carcinoma of the breast
Oncofetal antigens	
α_1-fetoprotein (AFP)	Hepatoma
	Testicular tumors
Carcinoembryonal antigen (CEA)	General
Hormones, enzymes, metal-binding proteins	
Human chorionic gonadotropin (β-HCG)	Chorionic carcinoma
	Testicular tumors
Parathormone (PTH)	Bronchogenic carcinoma
	Carcinoma of the pancreas
Adrenocorticotrophic hormone (ACTH)	Bronchogenic carcinoma
	Carcinoma of the pancreas
	Thymus tumors
Calcitonin	Carcinoma of the thyroid
	Bronchogenic carcinoma
Renin	Wilms' tumor
Casein	Carcinoma of the breast
Acid phosphatase	Carcinoma of the prostate
Alkaline phosphatase	Bone tumors (liver)
Tumor-specific antigens	

Melanoma, bronchogenic carcinoma, osteosarcoma, neuroblastoma, carcinoma of the breast etc.

In general, the detection of tumor-associated antigens has the following possible applications:

Early Diagnosis

Since the concentration of most tumor-associated antigens clearly increases only in the advanced stages of illnesses, it has not been previously possible to use them for early diagnosis of risk groups. Certain peptide hormones, that are already clearly elevated at the time of diagnosis, may prove to be an exception. First results indicate that they might be used for early diagnosis, for example, of bronchogenic tumors [8]. The detection of α_1-fetoprotein (AFP) in patients with liver cirrhosis is also suitable for early detection of hepatoma [6].

Diagnosis

Tumor-associated antigens that are characteristic for a certain tumor type are of diagnostic importance, e.g. AFP for hepatoma [6], AFP and β-HCG for teratomas [5], and ACTH for oat-cell carcinoma [4]. However, in general, the diagnostic value of tumor-associated antigens is minimal for the majority of tumors.

Tumor Localization

At the present, the same holds true for determining the localization of a tumor by means of antisera to certain tumor-associated antigens. This method, using total-body scintigraphy after administration of anti-CEA or anti-AFP, is still much too complex and costly, and it has by no means been proven to be superior to the conventional procedures.

Prognosis

An important area for detection of tumor-associated antigens is the evaluation of prognosis of tumor patients. This is true for such markers as CEA or ferritin; the serum concentrations of both closely correlate with the tumor mass, and their elevation signal either an incomplete resection or formation of metastases [1,7]. Adjuvant chemotherapy trials will most probably use tumor markers increasingly in the future to characterize high-risk groups.

Monitoring Disease

The most important area for the detection of tumor-associated antigens is monitoring the course of illness in order to detect early recurrences. Examples are the second-look operations of patients with increasing CEA serum levels, which previously have been operated for carcinoma of the colon [7], and additional treatment efforts in cases of testicular cancers [5], and oat-cell carcinomas [4] following an elevation of the corresponding marker.

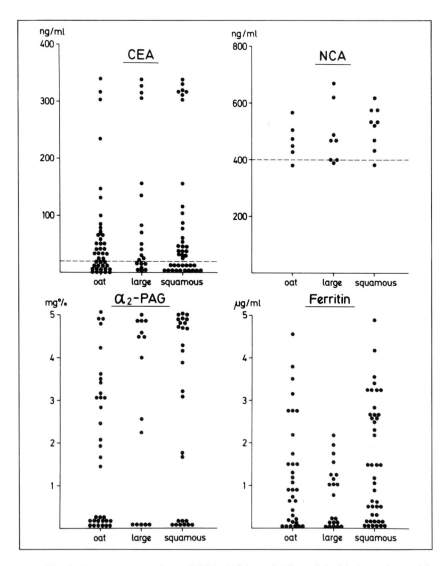

Fig. 1. Serum concentrations of CEA, NCA, α_2-PAG, and ferritin in patients with bronchogenic carcinoma.

In the following I will report on a number of our results in 2 groups of patients: patients with bronchogenic carcinoma and patients with malignant lymphomas. Moreover, I would like to draw attention to a special attempt of our study group: the analysis of antigens in circulating immune complexes. The characterization of these antigens may allow us to develop more specific immunologic procedures to detect the presence of tumors.

More than half of the patients with bronchogenic tumors (fig. 1) exhibit an elevated serum-level of the oncofetal antigen CEA, of NCA, of the pregnancy associated protein α_2-PAG, and of the iron-binding protein ferritin. Although no relationship has been found between these proteins and a certain histological tumortype, these proteins are especially elevated in metastatic disease. Figure 2 presents these data for CEA. Concerning the concentration of peptide hormones in the serum of patients with bronchogenic carcinoma, especially ACTH, calcitonin, parathormone, and β-HCG are elevated (fig. 3). In contrast to the previously cited proteins, these hormones are also increased in localized tumor forms. Moreover, ACTH and calcitonin are especially correlated to oat-cell carcinoma.

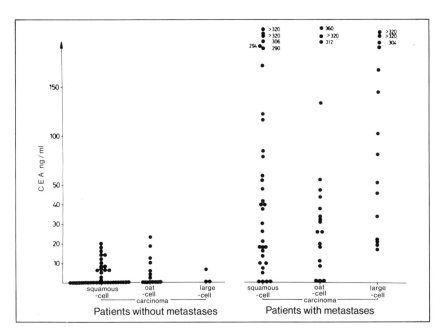

Fig. 2. CEA-serum levels in patients with bronchogenic carcinoma and in patients with and without metastases.

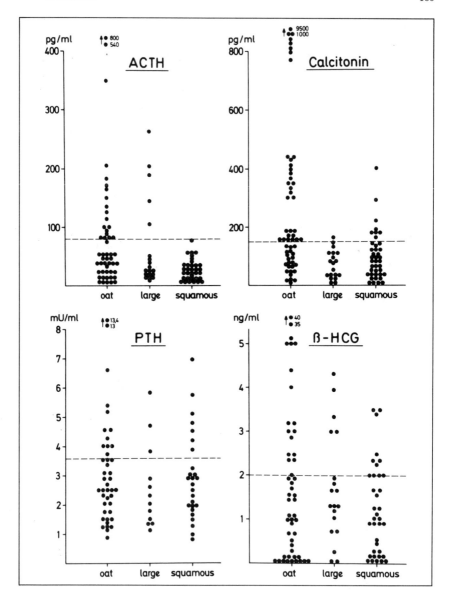

Fig. 3. ACTH, calcitonin, parathormone, and β-HCG in the serum of patients with bronchogenic carcinoma.

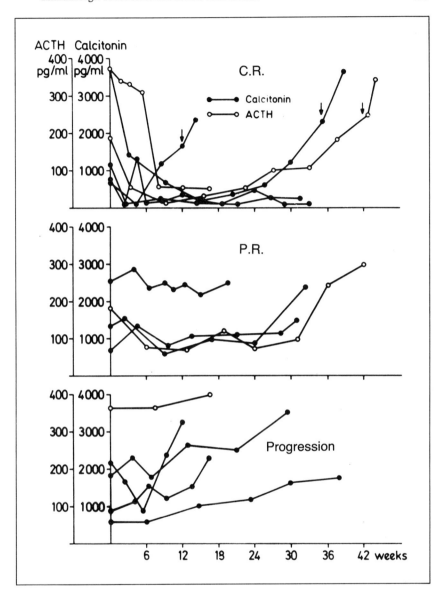

Fig. 4. Determination of ACTH and calcitonin serum levels during the course of polychemotherapy in patients with oat-cell carcinoma (arrows indicate clinical evidence of relapse).

Due to their frequent detection, even at the time of diagnosis, ACTH and calcitonin are particularly suitable for evaluating the course of disease of patients with oat-cell carcinoma (fig. 4). In case of complete remission, their concentrations regularly normalize. As long as the complete remission continues, the hormones also remain in the normal range. However, during recurrence, a continuous increase in concentration is often detected months before the recurrence is clinically evident. Conversely, in cases of partial remission, normal values are never observed, whereas during progression, the values of these hormones continue to rise.

As mentioned before, the detection of these proteins in the serum of tumor patients does not necessarily indicate that immune reactions, e.g. in the form of circulating antibodies, are directed against these substances. On the other hand, circulating immune complexes are elevated in the sera of patients with numerous tumor forms. Their detection is especially correlated to advanced disease and circulating immune complexes as well as tumor-associated antigens are suitable for evaluating the course of disease.

By employing 2 methods, circulating immune complexes are detected at diagnosis in 50% and 80% respectively of patients with bronchogenic carcinoma (fig. 5). In metastatatic disease, the frequency of detection amounts to 75–95%. During the course of the illness, the values normalize when a complete remission is achieved, whereas during progression, their concentration further rises. As a general rule, the levels of immune complexes increase again in case of recurrence.

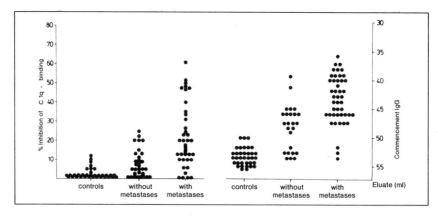

Fig. 5. Detection of circulating immune complexes in patients with bronchogenic carcinoma by 2 methods (C_{1q}-deviation and column chromatography).

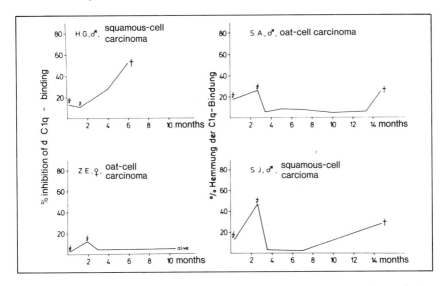

Fig. 6. Circulating immune complexes in patients with bronchogenic carcinoma during the course of disease.

A further interest of our study group was to characterize the antigens present in immune complexes of patients with oat-cell carcinoma. So, the macromolecular IgG fractions of patients with circulating immune complexes were separated by gradient centrifugation which then were further purified by binding to protein A (fig. 7). The purified immune-complex

Table II. C_{1q}-binding activity, tumor-associated antigens, and peptide hormones in sera of patients with oat-cell carcinoma

	C_{1q}-De-viation (%)	Ferritin µg/ml	α_2-PAG mg%	CEA ng/ml	ACTH pg/ml	Calcitonin pg/ml	PTH mU/ml
Normal levels up to	10	$\varnothing$	0.1	10	50	150	3.6
Patients							
He	18	5	3.5	19	70	430	2.2
S. W.	28	8	1.2	32	>800	400	3.5
Gb	12.5	12	0.8	45	40	380	2.5
Ro	17	3	2.6	150	90	220	7.9
Rh	29	4	1.9	21	6	62	3.0
Sch	26	4	1.3	30	12	62	2.8
Fr	13	1	2.2	57	100	120	2.3

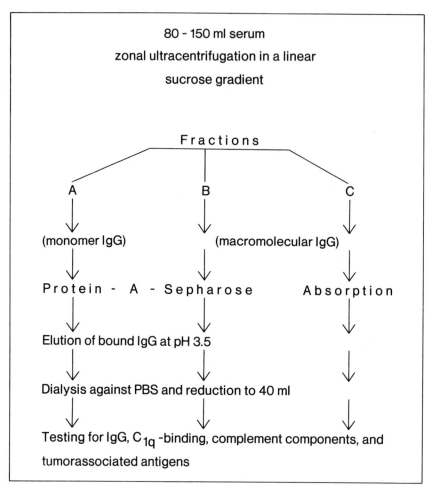

Fig. 7. Schematic presentation of the procedure for isolating immune complexes.

fractions were then tested for tumor-associated antigens present in the patients. Table II shows the tumor-associated antigens present in the patients' sera, whereas table III presents the results of these determinations in the isolated immune complexes. CEA, NCA, ferritin, α_2-PAG, alkaline phosphatase, and T-antigen were not present in the immune-complex fractions. In contrast, ACTH and, in some cases, also parathormone were detected in the immune-complex fractions. The characterization of the immune-complex-bound autoantigen ACTH shows that it

Table III: Concentration of C_{1q}-binding activity, protein, C4, ACTH and PTH (determined by radioimmunoassay and bioassay) in serum fractions of patients with bronchogenic carcinoma following zonal ultracentrifugation and protein A-Sepharose absorption chromatography

Patient	Fraction	C_{1q}-Deviation (%)	Protein ng/ml	IgG mg/ml	C_4	ACTH (RIA)* pg/ml	ACTH (bio-assay)**	PTH (RIA)*** mU/ml
He	A	∅	1.5	1.1	∅	∅	10	∅
	B	12.3	0.95	0.6	∅	350	40	1.6
	C	34.1	0.16	0.1	+	490	56	1.6
S. W.	A	∅	6.0	>2.0	∅	20	36	∅
	B	21.6	1.0	0.24	+	255	100	∅
	C	47	2.0	1.5	+	490	95	∅
Gb	A	∅	0.9	0.6	∅	∅	∅	∅
	B	12.3	0.45	0.26	∅	15	∅	∅
	C	15	0.08	0.12	∅	130	50	∅
Ro	A	∅	0.85	0.55	∅	∅	∅	∅
	B	18	0.78	0.4	+	10	20	0.5
	C	18.6	0.19	0.15	+	90	55	5.9
Rh	A	∅	0.7	0.6	∅	∅	∅	∅
	B	12	0.45	0.4	+	∅	∅	∅
	C	23.5	0.12	0.1	∅	∅	∅	∅
Sch	A	∅	2.0	1.6	∅	∅	∅	∅
	B	19	0.7	0.5	∅	40	∅	∅
	C	22	0.14	0.1	∅	∅	∅	∅
Fr	A	∅	1.2	0.9	∅	∅	∅	∅
	B	25	0.6	0.3	∅	∅	∅	∅
	C	18.4	0.1	0.08	+	∅	∅	∅

   * levels of > 50 pg/ml,
  ** % release of corticosteron in relation to controls, 50% or more and
*** levels of > 0.5 mU/ml were considered to be positive.

belongs to a group of glycoproteins with high molecular weight, probably representing the precursor molecules of ACTH. These precursor forms are produced by the tumor and released into the circulation. With the aid of a simple protein-A-binding method, IgG and immune complex IgG were obtained from the sera of a large number of patients, and ACTH and parathormone were determined in these IgG fractions (fig. 8). In the majority of patients with oat-cell carcinoma, ACTH and, in some instances, also parathormone were found to be present. In contrast, these hormones could not be detected in the protein-A fractions of sera from other types of tumor even when the sera indicated elevated ACTH values.

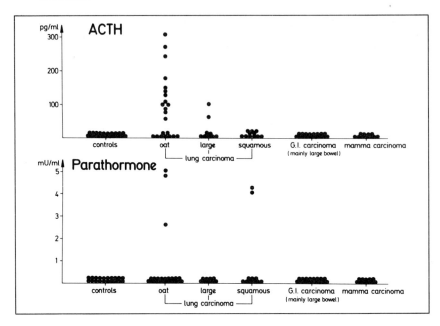

Fig. 8. Determination of immune complexes containing ACTH and parathormone (protein-A method) in healthy volunteers and patients with different tumors.

Thus, the detection of antigen-specific immune complexes will probably be of greater importance in the future than the detection of tumor-associated antigens, due to their higher specificity for the diagnosis of certain tumor forms. This will probably be also true for the detection of tumor antigens in tissue sections. Heterologous antisera to immune complexes containing ACTH and parathormone after absorption of anti-IgG and antibodies against complement components show a strong reaction with the tumor extracts from different bronchogenic carcinomas. Tumor cells containing these antigens could either be detected in tissues by means of immunofluorescence (fig. 9) or the immunoperoxydase method.

We also attempted to characterize the antigens in immune complexes of a second group of malignomas, the malignant lymphomas. Malignant lymphomas show circulating immune complexes particularly in the advanced stage and in the presence of B-symptoms. The immune complexes were isolated in a number of patients with Hodgkin's disease in the same way as it was carried out in patients with oat-cell carcinoma (see also fig. 7). These were then used to immunize rabbits. Subsequently the antisera

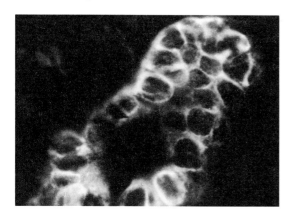

Fig. 9. Cytoplasmic and membrane fluorescence of tumor cells (oat-cell carcinoma; indirect immunofluorescence) with antisera against immune complexes of a patient with oat-cell carcinoma.

were exhaustively adsorbed in order to remove antibodies to IgG and complement components. Testing of the adsorbed antisera against Hodgkin sera with the Laurel electrophoresis showed a weak but obvious reaction. After the antisera were investigated by the immunoperoxydase method on lymph-node sections from patients with Hodgkin's disease, stained Sternberg Read cells and Hodgkin cells could be identified. Although we still have no results giving information on the nature of the antigen responsible, the selective demonstration of tumor cells in this disease shows that specific antigen detection may be possible by this method.

References

1   Chu, T. M.; Laven, P.; Day, J.; Evans, J. T.; Mittlemann, A.; Holoyoke, E. D.; Vincent, R.: Carcino-Embryonic Antigen: Prognosis and monitoring of cancer. In Lehmann (ed.), Carcino-Embryonic Proteins I, p. 55 (Elsevier, Amsterdam, 1979)
2   Goldenberg, D. M.; DeLand, F.; Euishin, K.; Bennett, S.; Primus, F. J.; van Nagell, J. R.; Estes, N.; DeSimone, P.; Rayburn, P.: Use of radiolabeled antibodies to carcinoembryonic antigen for the detection and localization of diverse cancers by external photoscanning. N. Engl. J. Med. *298:* 1384 (1978).
3   Havemann, K.: Immunstimulation in der Behandlung menschlicher Tumoren? Internistische Welt *9:* 306 (1979).
4   Havemann, K.; Gropp, C.: Ektope Hormonproduktion beim kleinzelligen Bronchialcarcinom. Biologische und immunologische Aspekte. Internist *21:* 84 (1980).
5   Javadpour, N.: The value of biologic markers in diagnosis and treatment of testicular cancer. Semin. Oncol. *6:* 37 (1979).
6   Lehmann, F.-G.; Wegener, T.: α-Fetoprotein in liver cirrhosis. II. Early detection of hepatoma. In Lehmann (ed.), Carcino-Embryonic Proteins I, p. 233 (Elsevier, Amsterdam 1979).

7   Mach, J. P.; Lamerz, R.: Postoperative surveillance and monitoring of cancer patients
     by sequential CEA immunoassays. In Lehmann (ed.), Carcino-Embryonic Proteins I,
     p. 83 (Elsevier, Amsterdam 1979).
8   Wilson, A. R.; Odell, W. D.: Pro-ACTH: Use for early detection of lung cancer. Am. J.
     Med. 66: 765 (1979).

Prof. Dr. K. Havemann, Medizin. Klinik am Klinikum der Philipps-Universität, Mann-
kopffstr. 1, D-3550 Marburg

Determination of Immune Complexes –
Its Significance for Clinical Oncology

G. Krieger, A. Kehl, M. Kneba, I. Bause

Med. Universitätsklinik, Abt. Hämatologie/Onkologie, Göttingen, FRG

An evaluation of the clinical significance of the detection of immune complexes for oncology should attempt to answer the following three question complexes:

(1) Can immune complexes be used as tumor markers that correlate closely with the tumor mass and that offer advantages over the other easily determined tumor markers or can they, together with these markers, supply additional information?

(2) Do the immune complexes have other biological importance surpassing that first mentioned, e.g., do they give information about the tumor host relationships and thus, independently of the tumor mass, supply information for the prognosis or even the response to a subsequent chemotherapy? Do clinical observations – not findings of animal experiments or results of in vitro tests – suggest such a role for the immune complexes and consequently the reasonable possibility of removing them by plasmapheresis or immunoabsorption?

(3) Finally, are there suitable methods of detecting immune complexes available in the clinic, i.e., can the relation between cost and usefulness be justified?

Despite the wealth of available data, the difficulty in answering these questions soon becomes apparent if one compares, for instance, the results of immune complex determinations in tumor patients with those in patients with systemic lupus erythematosis (SLE). Cases of SLE show good correlation between the course of the disease, especially with reference to nephritis and possibly also to cerebral involvement (of even greater importance for diagnosis), and the concentration of immune complexes in the serum. The different methods for detecting immune complexes also yield results that correlate, as the WHO study on methods of detecting immune complexes show (table I).

Findings in 23 patients with lupus erythematosis (LE) were almost identical when the Raji-cell test; the C_{1q} binding assay, and the C_{1q} solid-phase assay were used. Probably the most frequently applied tests, they also showed a very good correlation with each other [6].

Table I. Methods discriminating systemic lupus versus normal group

	% pos. *
RAJI	91
C_{1q}-BA	78
PAT2	74
PAT1	65
KIT	65
C_{1q}-SP**	58

* pos. = over 90th percentile ($p<0.05$ by χ^2 analysis for all methods listed)
** n = 12 for SLE

Table II. Results obtained by 18 methods on sera from patients with cancer

	Seminoma	Lymphoma	Nasopharyngeal carcinoma
C_{1q}-BA	1/7*	7/10	4/9
C_{1q}-SP	0/7	3/10	1/9
C_{1q}-DV	0/7	1/10	1/9
C_{1q}-LI	0/7	0/9	3/8
C_{1q}-RI	0/6	2/8	1/9
KgB-SP	1/4	1/10	1/4
mRF-I	2/7	1/10	1/9
mRF-RI	1/6	0/8	3/9
pRF-I	3/6	2/10	2/9
pRF-LI	0/7	1/9	4/9
RAJI	0/7	2/10	6/9
ROS-I	0/6	1/10	0/7
PAT1	1/7	2/10	5/9
PAT2	0/7	1/10	7/9
MA-UI	N.D.	3/7	0/7
KIT	1/7	2/10	0/9
NIT	2/7	4/10	6/9
BET	0/7	0/10	0/9

* no. positive (over 90th percentile)/no. tested.

In contrast, the situation is very different in the case of malignant tumors, where there is virtually no correlation. Table II shows that precisely in malignant lymphomas, in which immune complexes are frequently found, a pronounced discrepancy exists between the results of the Raji-cell test and the C_{1q} binding test. Thus, it is not surprising that a multitude of results have been reported on different tumors by different investigators, who use different methods for determining immune complexes.

There are, therefore, no generally valid answers which can be applied to clinical oncology. Thus, we are forced to deal with individual studies. We have chosen three well-known studies for discussion. Each emphasizes the clinical significance of determining immune complexes and, consequently, represents a positive selection.

Höffken et al. [4], in a frequently cited work, reported the determinitation of immune complexes in patients with cancer of the breast both before and 1 year after operation. Initially in 22 patients and later in an even larger patient population, they observed a correlation between the prognosis factor, involvement of the lymph nodes at the time of operation, and the concentration of immune complexes in plasma. Patients, who had negative lymph-node involvement at the time of operation, showed low concentrations of immune complexes before the operation, and these decreased after 1 year. In contrast, those patients with positive lymph-node involvement and those dying postoperatively within 22 months showed high concentrations of immune complexes from the very beginning, and these values decreased only minimally after 1 year (fig. 1). This data suggest that immune complexes are markers for clinically nonapparent tumor masses. In the clinician's mind, the question instantly arises whether determining immune complexes before and after operation can aid in deciding the pros and cons of an adjuvant chemotherapy following the operation.

When following the progress of a patient operated on for gastrointestinal carcinoma, the importance of CEA (carcinoembryonic antigen) is undisputed in its role as a parameter for the course of disease. According to *Staab and Anderer* [8] the additional determination of immune complexes, in this case of CEA-specific immune complexes, should yield additional information. This postulation is supported by the course of the disease in a 66-year-old patient who was operated on for adenocarcinoma of the coecum ($T_2N_1M_o$) (fig. 2). Shortly after the operation, the patient had moderately elevated CEA and CEA immune complex concentra-

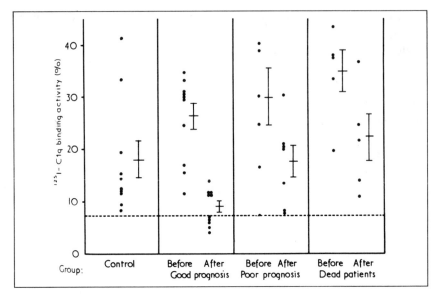

Fig. 1. Mean ^{125}J-C_{1q}-binding activities ($\pm$ S.E.) in women with breast cancer before and 12 months after mastectomy;
good prognosis = no lymph node involvement;
bad prognosis = metastases in lymph nodes at mastectomy;
dead patients = those who died from cancer within 22 months after the operation.

tions; these first decreased and then, to a large extent, increased again in parallel. The clinical consequence of a rise in the CEA-titer is the search for a relapse or metastases and eventually a second-look operation, as was carried out in this patient. The operation revealed liver metastases but no localized recurrence. Out of 37 patients subjected to second-look operations, 18 had CEA immune complexes. Of these, 16 showed presence of metastases; the 2 without metastases exhibited distant metastases at a later stage of the disease. Those patients who presented immune complexes already at the time of the first operation could, as a rule, only be treated palliatively due to the metastases. This investigation supports the usefulness of CEA immune complexes as markers for tumor masses that are growing but are clinically difficult to detect (e.g., occult metastases).

The investigations of *Nicole Carpentier* in cases of acute leukemia [1] advocate the additional biological significance of immune complexes, independently of tumor masses. She and her co-workers were able to show that patients with high concentrations of immune complexes responded less well to therapy than patients with no measurable titer of

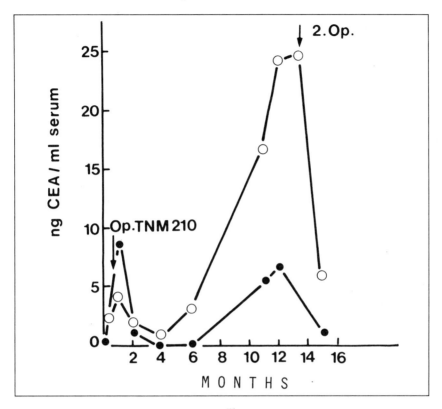

Fig. 2. Follow-up of an individual patient with excised adenocarcinoma of the coecum and second-look surgery by means of CEA (void circles) and CEA immune complexes (filled circles).

immune complexes; this finding was independent of age and of the diagnosis of acute myeloid or acute lymphatic leukemia (fig. 3). Moreover, the presence of immune complexes was independent of the number of lymphocytes and thrombocytes, bone-marrow infiltration, cytology, and blood sedimentation.

The most recent investigations by *Carpentier* [2] also revealed a clear dependence between positive findings of immune complexes and response to chemotherapy in cases of metastasizing carcinoma of the breast.

These studies not only support the clinical significance of immune complexes as markers for a clinically nonapparent tumor mass, carcinoma of the breast and colon, but also indicate that the immune complexes have a negative influence on tumor behavior such as the tumor's poor response

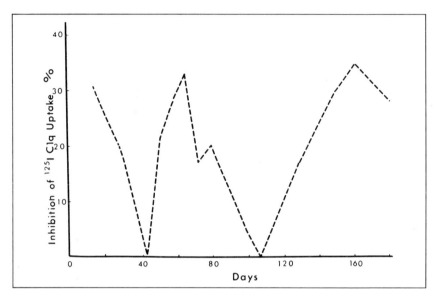

Fig. 3. The response rates in relation to the presence of immune complexes in various age groups of patients with AML and ALL: Patients with detectable circulating immune complexes at onset of leukemia are represented by the shaded columns and those without such complexes by the plain columns. In each column the dotted areas indicate the proportion of patients in whom the response to treatment was limited to partial remission.

to therapy, independent of the tumor mass. However, these results must be confirmed by other investigators, and the value of immune complex determinations must be examined critically within the framework of the other prognosis factors, especially with regard to cost and labor. This is especially true for carcinoma of the breast where, for example, the relation with hormone status has to be checked.

Since August 1980, we have examined 96 outpatients with metastasizing carcinoma of the breast by means of the C_{1q} binding assay according to *Nydegger* [7] as modified by *Zubler* [11]. A total of 26 of these patients (roughly one-fourth) showed positive findings. It is still too early for an evaluation of these findings, especially in relation to the course of the disease. Nevertheless, it is already possible to state that there is no correlation between clinically visible tumor masses with evident progression of the tumor and other factors such as blood sedimentation, CEA, and prolactin.

Further investigations of the course of the disease will reveal whether or not the immune complexes in these patients can predict a recurrence before the detection of CEA-titers, unphysiological blood sedimentation, and clinical picture; or if, when combined with an increase of CEA concentration and blood sedimentation, they can possibly predict a poor response to chemotherapy. However, it is equally possible that these tests in our patient material will show that the immune complexes have no clinical relevance.

Tests for the detection of immune complexes are quite costly, especially if the demand of the immunologists is met and several tests are carried out (table III).

Ideally a physical test (e.g., a chromatographic method) should be combined with a complement-dependent test (C_{1q} binding assay) and perhaps also with a Fc-receptor-dependent test (e.g., a rheumatoid-factor

Table III. Antigen-nonspecific methods for detecting circulating immune complexes

1. Physical techniques
   Analytical ultracentrifugation
   Sucrose density gradient centrifugation
   Gel filtration
   Ultrafiltration
   Electrophoresis
   Polyethylene glycol (PEG) precipitation
   Cryoprecipitation
2. Methods based on the biologic characteristics of immune complexes
   a) Complement techniques
      Microcomplement consumption test
      Assays based on the interaction of ICs with purified C_{1q} (C_{1q} precipitation in gels, C_{1q}-PEG test, C_{1q} deviation tests, C_{1q} solid-phase radioimmunoassays)
      Assays of breakdown products of C3 and C1
      The C3 precipitation assay
      The conglutinin radioimmunoassay
   b) Antiglobulin techniques
      Rheumatoid factor tests
      Other antiglobulin tests
   c) Cellular techniques
      The platelet aggregation test
      Inhibition of antibody-dependent cell-mediated toxicity
      Intracytoplasmic staining of polymorphonuclear leukocytes
      Release of enzymes from eosinophils and mast cells
      The macrophage inhibition assay
      Rosette inhibition tests
      The Raji-cell assay
      The L1210 murine leukemia cell assay
      The human erythrocyte assay
   d) Other methods
      Binding to staphylococcal protein A

test). Our own experience with the C_{1q} binding assay and the Raji-cell test according to *Theofilopoulos* [10], which we carried out as an immuno-fluoresence test or ELISA, shows how justified this demand is. Whereas in 3 patients, with SLE similarly high, concentrations of immune complexes were found in both tests, the agreement between the C_{1q} binding assay and the Raji-cell test is very poor in tumor patients. For example, one patient with carcinoma of the breast had the highest concentration of immune complexes in the Raji-cell test but a negative finding in the C_{1q}-binding assay. Conversely, one patient with bronchial carcinoma had the highest value in the C_{1q} binding assay but a negative result in the Raji-cell test. In addition, little is known about the dependence of the tests on blood sampling and storage of samples. Our experience has shown that the Raji-cell test is very sensitive to storage and one-time thawing, whereas the C_{1q} binding assay, under the same conditions, is considerably less sensitive.

In conclusion, it must be stated that as long as there is no other, simpler, antigen-specific procedure available, e.g., the procedure developed by *Havemann and Sedlaceck* [3] to detect Big-ACTH immune complexes, the determination of immune complexes must be reserved for scientific questions, especially if it can reveal the patient's course as depicted in figure 4. This figure shows the fluctuations of immune com-

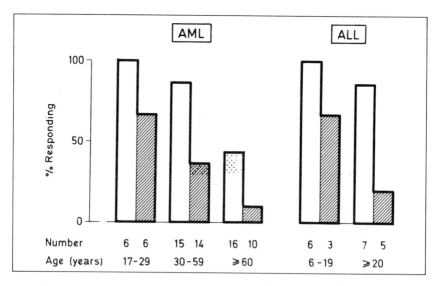

Fig. 4. Cyclic variation in C_{1q}-reactive material with time. Patient with stage II resected melanoma under treatment with oral BCG (120 mg weekly).

plexes in a patient with melanoma. The immune complexes were determined with a C_{1q} deviation test. The clinical course of the disease during the period of observation revealed no changes. In case of immune complex fluctuations, without depending on any clinical evidence, it should prove difficult to draw clinically relevant conclusions from either positive or negative determinations of immune complexes.

References

1   Carpentier, N. A.; Lange, G. T.; Fiere, D. M.; Fournie, G. J.; Lambert, P.-H.; Miescher, P. A.: Clinical relevance of circulating immune complexes in human leukemia. J. clin. Invest. *60:* 874–884 (1977).

2   Carpentier, N.; Chollet, P.; Betail, G.; Plagne, R.; Lambert, P. H.: Immune complexes: Escape mechanism of tumor cell in breast cancer? 4th International Congress of Immunology, Abstr.-No. 10.306 (Paris, July 1980).

3   Gropp, C.; Havemann, K.; Scheuer, A.; Gramse, M.: Studies of identification of antigens in immune complexes of lung-cancer patients. XII. Tagung der Gesellschaft für Immunologie, Abstr.-Nr. 46 (Garmisch-Partenkirchen, October 1980), Immunbiol. *157:* 3 (1980).

4   Höffken, K.; Meredith, J. D.; Robins, R. A.; Baldwin, R. W.; Davies, C. J.; Blamey, R. W.: Circulating immune complexes in patients with breast cancer. Br. med. J. *ii:* 218–220 (1977).

5   Jerry, L. M.; Rowden, G.; Cano, P. O.; Phillips, T. M.; Deutsch, G. F.; Capek, A.; Hartmann, D.; Lewis, M. G.: Immune complexes in human melanoma: A consequence of deranged immune regulation. Scand. J. Immun. *5:* 845–859 (1976).

6   Lambert, P. H.; Dixon, F. J.; Zubler, R. H.; Agnello, V.; Cambiaso, C. et al.: A WHO collaborative study for the evaluation of 18 methods for detecting immune complexes in serum. J. clin. Lab. Immunol. *1:* 1–15 (1978).

7   Nydegger, U. E.; Lambert, P. H.; Gerber, H.; Miescher, P. A.: Circulating immune complexes in the serum in systemic lupus erythematosus and in carriers of hepatitis-B-antigen. J. clin. Invest. *54:* 297–309 (1974).

8   Staab, H. J.; Anderer, F. A.; Stumpf, E.; Fischer, R.: Rezidivprognosen bei Patienten mit Adenocarcinomen des Gastrointestinaltraktes auf der Basis von carcinoembryonalem Antigen (CEA) und seinen zirkulierenden Immunkomplexen. Klin. Wschr. *58:* 125–133 (1980).

9   Theofilopoulos, A. N.; Dixon, F. J.: The biology and detection of immune complexes. Adv. Immunol. *28:* 89–220 (1979).

10 Theofilopoulos, A. N.; Wilson, C. B.; Dixon, F. J.: The Raji-cell radioimmunoassay for detecting immune complexes in human sera. J. clin. Invest. *57:* 169–182 (1976).

11 Zubler, R. H.; Lange, G.; Lambert, P. H.; Miescher, P. A.: Detection of immune complexes in unheated sera by modified J^{125}-C_{1q} binding test. J. Immun. *116:* 232–235 (1976).

Dr. G. Krieger, Medizinische Universitätsklinik, Abt. Hämatologie/Onkologie, Robert-Koch-Str. 40, D–3400 Göttingen

Bio-Assays as a Tool for the Demonstration of Immune Alteration in Cancer Patients: Suppression of Mitogen-Induced Lymphocyte Proliferation by Patients' Sera during Plasma Exchange – Preliminary Results in Four Patients –

P. Schuff-Werner[1, 3], N. Brattig[2], J.-H. Beyer[1, 3], J. Bartel[2], P. A. Berg[2], G. A. Nagel[1]

[1] Medizin. Universitätsklinik, Abt. Hämatologie/Onkologie, Göttingen, FRG
[2] II. Medizin. Universitätsklinik, Tübingen, FRG
[3] Supported by grants of the Fazit-Foundation

Introduction

In the last decade, several studies have shown that alterations of humoral and cellular immune functions play an important role in controlling tumor growth [13, 14, 21].

Besides intrinsic defects of lymphocyte subpopulations, especially of suppressor cells and natural killer cells [4, 22], serum-blocking factors (SBF) could be demonstrated in vitro which inhibit numerous immunological functions (extrinsic defect) [12].

These factors can suppress a variety of immunological in vitro assays, e.g. mitogenic- and allogeneic-induced lymphocyte stimulation, immunoglobulin production in vitro, the macrophage migration test, rosette formation as well as cellular cytotoxicity (see table I).

The immunosuppressive or immunoregulatory activity of some serum components, in particular immune complexes and acute-phase reactants, as well as mediators such as prostaglandins, chalones, and hormones could also be demonstrated [1, 2, 23, 25]. There is, however, little knowledge about serum-blocking factors of low molecular weight (lymphokines?),

Table I. Methods to measure different lymphocyte functions in vitro which can be altered by immunomodulating serum components

---

(1) *Lymphocyte-transformation test (T-cell functions)*
 – mitogen-induced lymphocyte proliferation (PHA/Con-A)
 – antigen-induced lymphocyte proliferation (PPD, tetanol, candida, mitochondrial extract of neurospora crassa, allogeneic cells)
(2) *Antibody synthesis in vitro (B-cell function)*
 – determination of supernatant immunoglobulin following polyclonal pokeweed-mitogen stimulation
 – Plaque-assay
(3) *Lymphocytotoxicity*
 – natural killer-cell activity
 – T-cell-mediated cytotoxicity
 – antibody-mediated cytotoxicity
(4) *Further functional tests*
 – T-rosette formation
 – T-colony formation
 – Con-A-induced T-suppressor cells
 – lymphokine-induced migration inhibition
 – leukocyte-adherance inhibition

---

which may have specific inhibitory functions [8]. At the moment they are not sufficiently defined, and so, selective elimination of those factors is not yet possible. The hypothesis that serum factors blocking immunological defense mechanisms can be removed by extended plasma exchange has led to the new concept of plasmapheresis in treating patients with advanced cancer [17].

It was the aim of our study to investigate whether or not in vitro bioassays are useful for the detection of SBF in the absence of other more specific methods.

Patients and Methods

107 samples of sera from 4 patients with advanced cancer, refractory to conventional therapy (see table II), were collected during the course of either a single plasma exchange or a series of several exchanges repeated at short intervals (exchange volume 2–5 l). The samples were stored at −20°C for further immunological investigation.

Methodological details of plasma exchange, especially on the substitution solutions used, are reported elsewhere [6].

Table II. Patients and their diagnosis: Variations of substitution and number of plasma exchanges

	Diagnosis	Number of plasma exchange treatments (in brackets)		Substitution
		serial PE	total of single PE's	
1. Pat. W., U.:	Advanced breast cancer with multiple metastasis	1	5	HA
2. Pat. B., H. J.:	Hypernephroid carcinoma with multiple metastasis	3	15	HA + γ-gl./FFP
3. Pat. L., M.:	Hodgkin's disease (IV B)	3	15	HA/HA + γ-gl./ FFP
4. Pat. B., G.:	Hodgkin's disease (IV B)	3	15	FFP, FFP, HA

Immunological Methods

(1) Mitogen-Induced Lymphocyte-Transformation Test (LTT) for the in Vitro Demonstration of Serum-Blocking Factors

The lymphocyte-transformation test for the detection of SBF was carried out as described by *Berg* and *Brattig* (1976) [5].

Mononuclear peripheral blood cells were isolated from heparinized venous blood of healthy donors with Ficoll gradient centrifugation (Lymphoprep®) using the method of *Bøyum* (1968) [7].

After three washes in Hank's balanced salt solution (HBSS) the cells were adjusted to 2×10^5 cells in 0,2 ml culture medium (RPMi 1640) containing 20% heat-inactivated serum or plasma. Triplicates were cultured in a CO_2-enriched humidified atmosphere for 48 h. During the last 8 h of culture the lymphocytes were labeled with 3H-thymidine and then harvested with a semi-automatic cell-harvester (Skatron® cell harvester) on glass fiber filters (Whatman GF/C). The dried filters were counted in a liquid scintillation counter (Tricarb 3375). The results are given in counts per minute (cpm). The suppressive effect of patients' sera on the mitogen-induced proliferation of lymphocytes from normal donors as measured by 3H-thymidine incorporation was expressed as % inhibition calculated as follows:

$$\% \text{ Inhibition} = (1 - \frac{\text{cpm (test)}}{\text{cpm (control)}}) \cdot 100$$

(2) Inhibition of Antigen-Induced Lymphocyte Stimulation
Lymphocytes were prepared, cultured, and evaluated as described above. A pool of different recall antigens (50 μg purified protein derivative (PPD), 20 μg mitochondrial extract of neurospora crassa and tetanol 1 : 1000) was used for stimulation in a six-day culture.

(3) Determination of Immune Complexes
Immune complex levels in patients' sera were evaluated by C_{1q}-binding assay. The binding of FITC-labeled anti-human-IgG was determined by quantitative immunofluorescence as modified by *Bartel* and *Berg* [3]. C_{1q}-coated acetate foils were incubated over 30 min with patients' sera, washed and incubated with the fluorescein-conjugated anti-human IgG. After rewashing, evaluation was performed with a computerized fluorimeter (system Fiax-Stiq®, Boehringer/Ingelheim Diagnostik GmbH) and values are expressed as μg-aggregated IgG.

(4) Acute-Phase Reactants
($\alpha2$-macroglobulin, haptoglobin, $\alpha1$-antitrypsin) were determined by commercially available kits (Mancini-technique).

(5) The Calculation of Statistical Regression
was assessed with a Nova III calculator (Data General) using our own statistical program[1]. Conventional correlation coefficients, Spearman rank correlation coefficients and the regression-curves x (y) and y (x) were calculated.

Results

To test the influence of the human albumin used in substitution solutions during plasmapheresis, the responder cells of healthy donors were stimulated by 5 μg PHA in the presence of 20% albumin and normal

---

[1] The statistical evaluations were kindly provided by W. Schultz, physics study group in the Department of Nuclear Medicine, University Clinic Goettingen.

donor serum (mixed 1 : 1). Cultures were also run with either 20% pure albumin or normal donor serum alone.

A lack of nutritive serum factors may explain the 30% inhibition of PHA-induced blast transformation when the cells were only cultured in human albumin. Human albumin and normal serum at a ratio of 1 : 1 were not inhibitory when compared to the serum controls of normal donors (fig. 1).

Sera from two patients with Hodgkin's disease (IV b), taken before plasma exchange, did not inhibit the mitogenic stimulation of normal lymphocytes, whereas sera from a patient with breast cancer and a patient with hypernephroid carcinoma did suppress the 3H-thymidine incorporation by up to 50% as compared to control sera.

As shown in figure 2, the inhibitory activity was no longer detectable directly after the first plasma exchange, but 48 h later 5 out of 8 sera were again suppressive. At the end of each further exchange none of the sera inhibited the mitogen-induced lymphocyte stimulation.

Serum from the patient with breast cancer, taken just before plasma exchange, significantly suppressed the PHA-induced blast transformation to a range of 50%; the antigen-induced lymphocyte stimulation was suppressed by up to 95% using the same serum. After plasma exchange inhibition of mitogen stimulation was no longer observed and remained so during the further course of treatment. The inhibition of the antigen stimulation, however, could not be eliminated even by repeated exchanges (fig. 3).

Such a dissociation of the inhibitory behavior was not observed in a patient with hypernephroid carcinoma: the initially demonstrated inhibitory activity could be eliminated during serial plasma exchange (fig. 4).

As mentioned above, the sera of two patients with Hodgkin's disease (IV b) showed no inhibitory activity at the beginning of serial plasma exchange. 24 h after the second PE of a series of four PE's, there was about 40% suppression of PHA-induced lymphocyte transformation, which could be eliminated by a further exchange. However, 24 h later there was even an stronger inhibitory activity than before (fig. 5). This behavior of serum inhibitory activity was identical in both patients. The patients with Hodgkin's disease underwent a total of three serial treatments with plasma exchange under quasi identical conditions. During the first series they were only substituted with human albumin salt solution, whereas at the end of the second series with human albumin, high doses of gammaglobulin were applied.

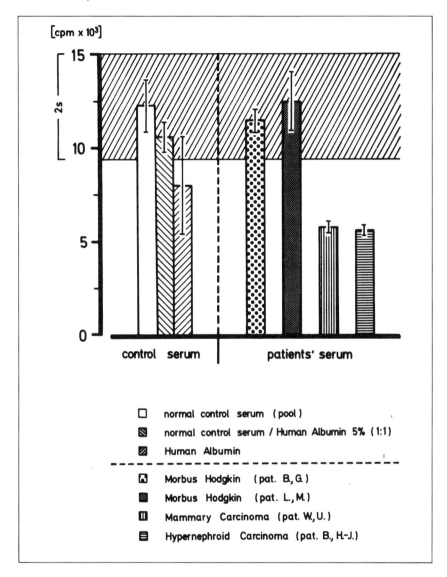

Fig. 1. Mitogen (5 µg PHA)-induced proliferation of lymphocytes from a normal donor cultured in the presence of patients' and control serum.

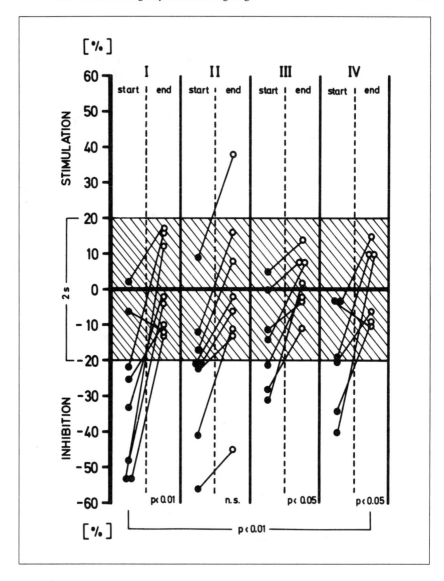

Fig. 2. Serial plasma exchange in tumor patients. Serum inhibitory activity before and after each exchange.

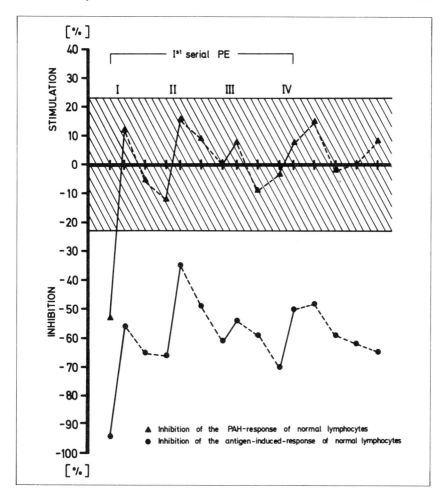

Fig. 3. PE in a patient with advanced breast cancer: Dissociation of the serum inhibitory activity evaluated by the mitogeneic and antigenic stimulation of normal lymphocytes.

The third series of plasma exchanges was performed with fresh frozen plasma (FFP).

After the last plasmapheresis in the first and third series there was an increase in serum inhibitory activity. In contrast after substitution with gammaglobulins (total doses 17.5 g), we were unable to demonstrate any significant inhibition of the PHA-stimulated normal lymphocytes (fig. 6).

Potential correlation, between the inhibition and both the level of

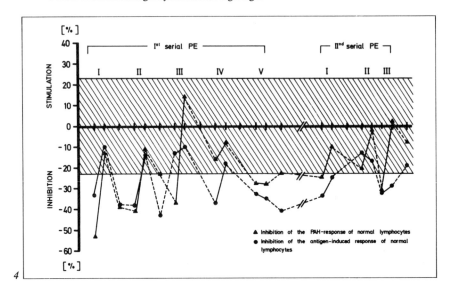

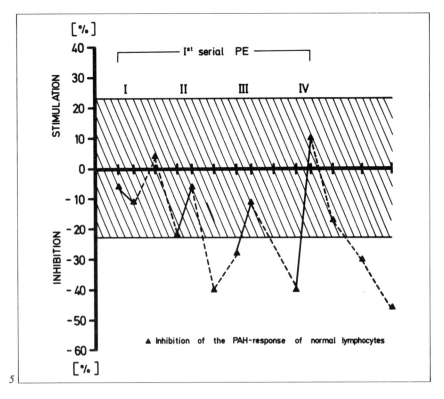

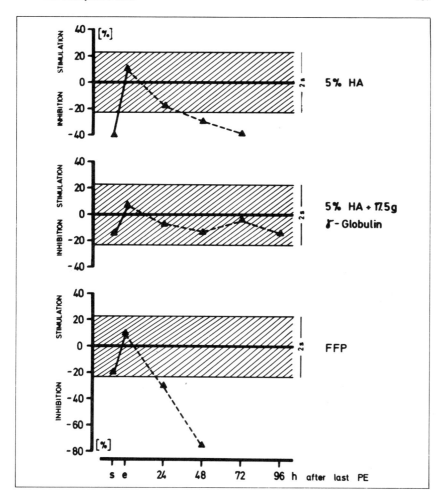

Fig. 6. Influence of different substitutes on the behavior of serum inhibitory activity after serial plasma exchange in a patient with Hodgkin's disease (IV B).
HA: Human albumin
FFP: Fresh frozen plasma

◁   *Fig. 4.* Serum inhibitory activity in the course of two plasma exchange series in a patient with advanced hypernephroid carcinoma.
        Fig. 5. Serum inhibitory activity in the course of serial plasma exchange in a patient with Hodgkin's disease (IV B).

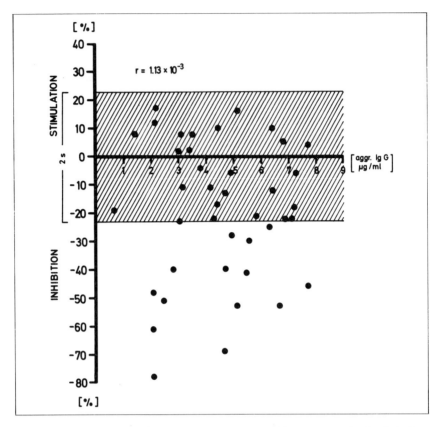

Fig. 7. Correlation of serum inhibitory activity and immune complex levels in four patients with advanced tumor disease during plasma exchange
(normal range: 3–7 µg aggr. IgG/ml).

immune complexes in the tested sera as well as other plasma components that interfered with immunoregulation, was tested for. No positive correlation ($r < 1.13 \times 10^{-3}$) was observed between inhibitory activity and the levels of immune complexes as far as they are detectable with our method. Correlations between the distinct tumor and plasma components showed that possibly α2-macroglobulin levels correlate with the serum inhibition (fig. 7).

The suppressing factors in the sera of our Hodgkin's disease patients correlate with changes of acute-phase reactant levels, especially of α1-antitrypsin and haptoglobin (fig. 8 and 9).

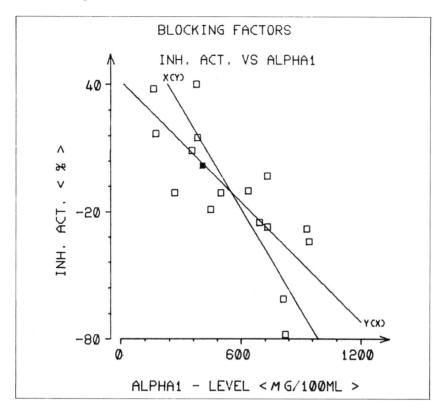

Fig. 8. Serial plasma exchange in a patient with Hodgkin's disease (IV B). Correlation of serum inhibitory activity to α1-antitrypsin level of the sera investigated (n = 17).
$r = -0,77$ (conventional regression coefficient)
$r_{sp} = -0,84$ (Spearman rank correlation coefficient)

Discussion

Our preliminary data, which must be treated with some reservation, indicate that it is possible to detect serum-blocking factors during the course of plasma-exchange treatment by in vitro assays, although it is not certain if such in vitro conditions are comparable to those in vivo.

We were also interested as to whether or not the grade of inhibition correlated with the levels of known immunosuppressive serum components such as acute-phase reactants (α2-macroglobulin, haptoglobin, α1-antitrypsin, transferrin, coeruloplasmin etc.) and immune complexes.

The investigations in the patient with advanced breast cancer and in

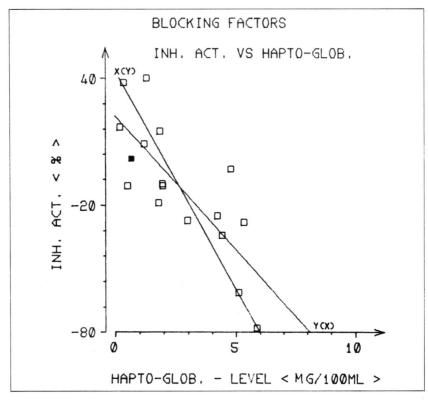

Fig. 9. Serial plasma exchange in a patient with Hodgkin's disease (IV B). Correlation of serum inhibitory activity to haptoglobin level of the sera investigated (n = 17).
r = −0,78 (conventional regression coefficient)
r_{sp} = −0,79 (Spearman rank correlation coefficient)

the patient with hypernephroid carcinoma allow the conclusion that immunosuppressive factors can be eliminated by serial plasma exchange. The reappearance of SFB after PE and the characterization of these factors are subjects of further investigations.

Antigen-antibody complexes ('immune complexes') play, both in vivo and in vitro, an immunoregulative role [10, 15, 20, 25]. In particular they may block cytotoxic reactions [12, 25] although it is still not certain as to whether or not this is an epiphenomenon related to the in vitro immunosuppression [15].

Immune complexes, as far as they are detectable by our method, seem to play no immunosuppressive role in the patients investigated: the few sera with low to moderately elevated immune complex levels were not identical to those sera producing strongest inhibition. It is difficult to interpret the finding that there appears to be a serum factor blocking PHA-stimulation, which can be removed by PE and a separate factor which affects antigen-induced lymphocyte stimulation and which is not eliminated on serial plasmapheresis. Besides such speculation about a second inhibitory factor, it must also be considered that perhaps specific antibodies can bind the stimulating antigens in the test assay or that they may form potentially inhibitory antigen-antibody-complexes. However, if this is so, it is surprising that the inhibition is always of a constant degree, since under the conditions of PE an increasing dilution of antibody titers must occur which causes the inhibitory activity to decrease continuously.

In two patients with Hodgkin's disease serum-mediated suppression of the described test system was not detectable at the beginning of PE, but increased after the second and following PE treatments. This immunosuppressive activity correlates statistically with the level of acute-phase reactants such as α1-antitrypsin and haptoglobin. Both substances are known to be immunosuppressive in vitro [2, 19]. The rapid increase in these sialoglycoproteins may reflect an unfavorable prognosis. Furthermore, it seems to be interesting that no serum inhibition could be detected during the same observation time when patients were given high doses of gammaglobulins at the end of PE; this phenomenon must however be shown to be reproducible in other patients before further speculation is allowed. It is imaginable that intact immunoglobulin molecules can block the rebound-phenomenon of rapid reproduction of serum inhibitors by binding to Fc-receptors of mediator-producing cells [24].

Conclusion

The inhibition of the mitogen- and antigen-induced lymphocyte-stimulation test may serve in the detection of blocking factors in sera of cancer patients under treatment with plasmapheresis.

Factors influencing the PHA-induced lymphocyte stimulation can be removed by plasmapheresis. As the preliminary results in four patients suggest, these inhibitory factors do not seem to correlate with immune complexes, but there are statistical hints for a correlation with acute-phase reactants.

The increase of inhibitory serum activity, in patients with Hodgkin's disease under plasmapheresis, is statistically correlated to a rise of acute-phase reactants (haptoglobin and α1-antitrypsin). This may be an expression of a prognosticly unfavorable stituation.

It seems to be of interest, that substitution with high doses of gammaglobulin depresses the recurrence of inhibitory activity after plasmapheresis in patients with Hodgkin's disease.

These preliminary results must be confirmed by further investigations in other patients.

References

1 Arora, P. K.; Miller, H. C.; Aronson, L. D.: α_1-antitrypsin is an effector of immunological stasis. Nature 274: 589–590 (1978).

2 Bata, J.; Cordier, G.; Revillard, J.-P.; Bonneau, M.; Latour, M.: Modulation of lymphocyte responses by serum protease-antiprotease systems. In: Touraine et al. (eds.), Transplantation and Clinical Immunology XI, pp. 59–70 (Excerpta Medica Amsterdam, Oxford, Princeton 1980).

3 Bartel, J.; Maier, E.; Maisch, B.; Berg, P. A.: Nachweis von Immunkomplexen in Seren von Patienten mit Leber- und Kollagenerkrankungen mittels eines fluorimetrischen Solidphase C_{1q}-Assays (FIAX). Kongreß für Laboratoriumsmedizin, Berlin, 3.–7. 5. 1981.

4 Blair, P. B.; Lane, M. A.: Non-T-cell killing of mammary tumor cells by spleen cells: Secretion of antibody and recruitment of cells. J. Immunol. 115: 184–189 (1975).

5 Brattig, N.; Berg, P. A.: Serum inhibitory factors (SIF) in patients with acute and chronic hepatitis and their clinical significance. Clin. exp. Immunol. 25: 40–49 (1976).

6 Beyer, J.-H.; Klee, M.; Bartsch, H.-H.; Borghardt, J.; Brockmeyer, J.; Kaboth, U.; Köstering, H.; Bolling, R.; Nagel, G. A.: First experiences with plasmapheresis in patients with neoplastic diseases. XV. German Cancer Congress, Munich, March 11–15, 1980 (abstract in press).

7 Böyum, A.: Isolation of mononuclear cells and granulocytes from human blood. Scand. J. clin. Lab. Invest. 21 (Suppl. 97): 77–89 (1968).

8 Cohen, S.; David, J.; Feldman, M.; Glade, P. R.; Mayer, M.; Oppenheim, J. J.; Papermaster, B. W.; Pick, E.; Pierce, C. W.; Rosenstreich, D. L.; Waksman, B. H.: Current state of studies of mediators of cellular immunity: A progress report. Cell. Immunol. 33: 233–244 (1977).

9 Goodwin, J. S.: Modulation of Con-A-induced suppressor cell activation by prostaglandin E_2. Cell. Immunol. 49: 421–425 (1980).

10 Gorczynski, R. M.; Kolburn, D. G.; Knight, R. A.: Nonspecific and specific immunosuppression in tumor-bearing mice by soluble immune complexes. Nature 254: 141–143 (1975).

11 Hellström, I.; Hellström, K. E.; Sjögren, H. O.; Warner, G. A.: Demonstration of cell-mediated immunity to human neoplasms of various histological types. Int. J. Cancer 7: 1–16 (1971).

12 Hellström, I.; Hellström, K. E.; Sjögren, H. O.; Warner, G. A.: Serum factors in tumor-free patients cancelling the blocking of cell-mediated tumor immunity. Int. J. Cancer 8: 185–191 (1971).

13 Herberman, R. B.: Cell-mediated immunity to tumor cells. Adv. Cancer Res. *19:* 207–263 (1974).
14 Herberman, R. B.: Immunologic tests in diagnosis of cancer. Am. J. clin. Path. *68:* 688–698 (1977).
15 Höffken, K.; Schmidt, C. G.: Immunkomplexe bei malignen Erkrankungen: Tumormarker oder Epiphänomen? Dt. med. Wschr. *105:* 1697–1699 (1080).
16 Houch, J. C.: Lymphocyte chalone. J. reticuloendoth. Soc. *24:* 571 (1978).
17 Israel, L.; Edelstein, R.; Mannoni, P.; Radot, E.; Greenspan, E. M.: Plasmapheresis in patients with disseminated cancer: Clinical results and correlation with changes in serum protein. Cancer (Philadelphia) *40:* 3146–3154 (1977).
18 Israel, L.; Edelstein, R.: In vivo and in vitro studies on nonspecific blocking factors of host origin in cancer patients: Role of plasma exchange as an immunotherapeutic modality. J. med. Soc. *14:* 105–130 (1978).
19 Johannsen, R.; Carlsson, A. B.; Haupt, H.; Heide, K.: Human-Blutproteine mit Hemmwirkung auf die Lymphozytentransformation in vitro. Behring Inst. Mitt. *54:* 33–44 (1974).
20 Kaattari, S.; Scibienski, R. J.; Benjamini, E.: The immunoregulatory role of antigen-antibody complexes: I. Assessment of B- and T-cell responses. Immunology *40:* 9–16 (1980).
21 Kamo, I.; Friedman, H.: Immunosuppression and the role of suppressive factors in cancer. Adv. Cancer Res. *25:* 271–321 (1977).
22 Kirchner, H.: Suppressor cells of immune reactivity in malignancy. Eur. J. Cancer *14:* 453–459 (1978).
23 Plescia, O. J.; Smith, A. H.; Grinwich, K.: Subversion of immune system by tumor cells and role of prostaglandins. Proc. natn. Acad. Sci. USA *72:* 1848–1851 (1975).
24 Schwenk, H.-U.; Baenkler, H.-W.: Effect of gammaglobulin injection on circulating immune complexes in various diseases. Eur. J. Paediat. *131:* 43–48 (1979).
25 Sjögren, H. O.; Hellström, I.; Bansal, S. C.; Hellström, K. E.: Suggestive evidence that the 'blocking antibodies' of tumor-bearing individuals may be antigen-antibody complexes. Proc. natn. Acad. Sci. USA *68:* 1372–1375 (1971).

Dr. P. Schuff-Werner, Medizin. Universitätsklinik, Abt. Hämatologie/Onkologie, Robert-Koch-Str. 40, D-3400 Göttingen

IV. Therapeutical Aspects of Plasma Exchange in Cancer Patients

Chairmen:
H. Borberg and *G. A. Nagel,* Göttingen

Repeated Plasma Exchanges in Patients with Metastatic Cancer

Lucien Israel, Richard Edelstein, Raymond Samak

Immunotherapy Unit, Hôpital Avicenne, University Paris XIII, Bobigny, France

Introduction

Sera from cancer patients possess the capacity to inhibit the blastogenic responses of normal lymphocytes to phytohemagglutinin [20]. This immunosuppressive effect of serum from cancer patients has since been widely confirmed in a variety of tumors and been used in several different in vitro models of immune function [5, 15, 17, 19].

The nature of the 'blocking factors' responsible for this effect is not known. Broadly speaking two categories of putative blocking factors have been suggested: those produced by the tumor itself, and those produced by the host in response to the presence of the tumor.

Among the former, blocking activity have been ascribed to free-tumor antigen [4], antigen-antibody complexes [21], and diverse polypeptides [23].

In addition to tumor products, the tumor-bearing host synthesizes a number of proteins, mostly α-globulins, in excessive quantities and it has been shown that these proteins, referred to collectively as acute-phase reactants, can exert immunosuppressive properties both in vivo and in vitro [3, 11, 14].

These reports appeared to us to provide a sufficiently strong rationale for attempting to remove blocking factors by the empirical approach of plasma exchange.

Material and Methods

Fifty-two patients with advanced metastatic cancer underwent plasma exchange. Of these, 2 had no evaluable disease and 5 did not complete the scheduled program (1 sudden death due to acute adrenal necrosis; 1 pulmonary embolism; 1 severe infection; 1 case of rapid aggravation of decompensated ascites and pleural effusion; and 1 preterminal case who went into coma). Thus 45 patients were evaluable for response. The primary sites included 14 melanoma, 6 breast, 5 kidney, 5 colon, 3 lung, 3 stomach, 3 fibrosarcomas, 2 thyroid and 1 each for head and neck, lymphosarcoma, teratoma and unknown primary.

4–5 l plasma exchanges were performed on a Haemonetics model 30 blood-cell separator. The procedure has been described in detail elsewhere [9].

The plasma substitute used was initially pooled human fresh-frozen plasma (FFP). The last 7 patients received both FFP and modified fluid gelatin with a view to reducing the amount of FFP required and hence the risk of viral hepatitis, and also to diminish the amount of plasma protein reinjected to the patient.

Initially the number of plasma exchanges was arbitrarily set at 2 a week and was subsequently increased to 3 a week after it was shown that a number of immunosuppressive acute-phase proteins depleted by plasma exchange returned to pretreatment levels within 48 h [11]. The number of sessions was initially 3 to 6 and was subsequently increased to 9 and even to 12 in 3 patients.

Routine biological tests were performed on all patients and, in addition, all patients underwent some or all of the following immunological tests prior to plasma exchange, immediately after the last session, and two weeks thereafter, in an attempt to demonstrate a correlation between an immunological profile and clinical response: quantitation of the acute-phase proteins haptoglobin, orosomucoid, fibrinogen, α_1-antitrypsin, transferrin, and ceruloplasmin; immunoglobulins IgG, IgA and IgM, complement components C3 and C4; B and T cell counts, lymphocyte blastogenesis to PHA, skin tests to PPD, candida and streptokinase, and in vivo macrophage migration by the Rebuck skin window technique. During plasma exchange, and for at least two weeks thereafter, patients received no other therapy. Subsequently each patient was treated by chemotherapy or chemoimmunotherapy according to the physician's best judgment.

Results

(a) Clinical Results

Of the 45 evaluable patients, 14 (31%) had an objective partial reduction in tumor mass, exceeding 50% (product of two perpendicular diameters); 12 (26%) had no change, and 19 (43%) had progressive disease. When patients responded they did so within 2–3 weeks of the last exchange session. Responses were seen most often in breast cancer (5/6), least often in melanoma (1/14). The other responding tumors were colon carcinomas (3/5), hypernephroma (2/5), thyroid carcinomas (2/2), and stomach cancer (1/3). The case histories of these patients have been described in detail elsewhere [9, 12].

After completion of the plasma exchange and the two to three week 'rest' period, patients were treated by chemotherapy or combined chemoimmunotherapy. Striking differences emerged in response rates to subsequent treatment between patients who responded initially to plasma exchange and those who did not. Of the 14 patients who had a partial response to plasma exchange, 8 had a partial or complete response to subsequent chemotherapy or chemoimmunotherapy (57%). By comparison, the response rates to subsequent treatment in patients who had no change or whose disease continued to progress after plasma exchange were 25% (3/12) and 11% (2/19) respectively. Median survival of plasma exchange responders from the time of the first plasma exchange was 12 months, versus 6 months for 'no change' patients and 3 months for progressors. The two longest survivors in each group are 63+ and 54; 24 and 12; 14 and 7 months respectively.

(b) Toxicity

Two fatalities occurred during the plasma exchange program. One patient died of hemorrhagic destruction of both adrenal glands and the second patient succumbed to a massive pulmonary embolism (this patient had a fibrosarcoma of the lung with extension to the pericardium and right atrium).

Viral hepatitis developed in 4 patients including one fatality. No cases of hepatitis have been seen in the last 24 patients. Assay for HBs antigen is performed every two months in the follow-up of these patients. Other moderate side effects included hypotension at the end of the extraction period, allergic reactions, and manifestations of hypocalcemia. These were easily managed by fluid replacement, antihistaminics or hydrocortisone and calcium gluconate respectively. No coagulation disturbances were seen. Platelet counts dropped by 50 % in virtually all patients but this was never of clinical consequence and pre-treatment levels were restored by the 10th day following the last exchange.

Immunological Parameters

Immunological parameters were examined for the population as a whole and separately for clinical responders and non-responders. A significant (student's paired t test) drop in the acute-phase proteins haptoglobin, orosomucoid, fibrinogen, and α_1-antitrypsin was observed immediately following the last exchange. After two weeks of post-treatment, levels returned to pre-treatment levels. No difference was noted between clinical responders and non-responders with regard to these protein changes.

A similar pattern was seen for the complement components C3, while C4 dropped significantly *in responders only*. Interestingly, pretreatment levels of C4 were significantly ($p < 0.01$) higher in responders and may therefore constitute a predictor for response.

Among the immunoglobulins, only IgG showed a significant change (decrease) and here again only in the group of clinical responders.

Assays for T- and B-lymphocytes and PHA-induced lymphocyte blastogenesis showed irregular changes following plasma exchange and no correlation could be established with the clinical response.

Skin tests to the recall antigens PPD, candida, and streptokinase were performed in 42 patients. 26 had an unchanged response following plasma exchange, 11 had an enhanced response and 5 had a weaker response. None of these changes correlated with the clinical result of the procedure.

In vivo macrophage migration, assayed by a modified version of the Rebuck skin window technique [18] was performed in 15 patients and revealed interesting results. Of the two clinical responders tested, both had a strikingly enhanced macrophage response following plasma exchange in terms of the number of macrophages migrating into an inflammatory site (< 1000 pretreatment versus 7500 and 10000 posttreatment). Two weeks later values returned to pretreatment levels. This pattern was seen in only 2/13 clinical non-responders.

Discussion

It is of considerable theoretical and practical interest that plasma exchange, used as a single treatment modality, has been able to produce objective regression in patients with an overwhelming tumor burden. This may signify that even in far advanced cancer, the immune system is not irrevocably destroyed but simply 'inhibited' and capable of being restored given the right conditions.

Indeed, plasmapheresis has been noted [7] to improve direct cell-mediated cytotoxicity in autologous serum and to increase the capacity of T-lymphocytes to form E-rosettes [2]. Another line of evidence for the reversibility of depressed lymphocyte function in cancer patients is that in vitro washing of these cells improves their responsiveness to the mitogen phytohemagglutinin [16].

The nature of the blocking factors removed by plasma exchange remains hypothetical. Our personal studies have indicated that a number of acute-phase proteins are markedly elevated in cancer patients irrespective of primary site, that the degree of elevation correlates well with the extent of disease [10], and that some of these proteins, particularly haptoglobin and fibrinogen, inhibit PHA-induced blastogenesis of normal lymphocytes and chemotaxis of normal monocytes [13, 14].

Circulating immune complexes between tumor antigen and specific antibody may also participate in the 'blocking' effect of cancer patients sera. Indeed, high titers of such complexes have been reported in cancer patients [6, 8] and their removal by immunoadsorption of serum over staphylococcal protein A (which selectively binds IgG and IgG-containing complexes) was reported to produce an objective clinical response in a patient with colon carcinoma [1] and dramatic necrosis of breast tumors in dogs [22]. It is interesting that our results showed decreased levels of IgG following plasma exchange only in patients who responded clinically to the procedure and this may reflect indirectly the effective clearance of immune complexes which we did not evaluate directly.

For reasons that are not clearly understood, patients whose tumors regressed partially after plasma exchange had a markedly improved response to subsequent chemoimmunotherapy as compared to patients who did not respond to plasma exchange, and their survival was significantly prolonged. Of all the patients with metastatic cancer referred for plasma exchange only three survived beyond 4 years and all three showed objective regression following the procedure. This observation considerably increases the benefit derived from plasma exchange which was initially thought to be only transient.

From the patient population treated so far it has emerged that malignant melanoma is a poor indication for plasma exchange (one responder out of 14 patients) while the most promising results have been achieved in breast cancer (5/6 objective regressions). It is still too early to define rigidly the indications for the procedure and further screening will determine whether certain types of tumors are more suitable than others.

When this study began, plasma exchange was performed twice or three times weekly and the exchange volume was 4 to 5 l. Since then we have shown that immunosuppressive acute-phase proteins are rapidly renewed after plasma exchange [11] and that similar rapid renewal occurs for immune complexes. Further, with each cycle of exchange, some of the replacement fluid administered for preceding cycles is of necessity withdrawn and hence the *effective volume of patient's removed plasma* diminishes with each successive cycle. These considerations have led us to initiate a new protocol in March 1980 using smaller (2 l) and more frequent (daily) exchanges.

As for all new procedures, plasma exchange has been tested in patients with very advanced disease and this raises the same problems as with other previously unproven modalities. If plasma exchange alone can produce regression of an overwhelming tumor burden, might it not be of greater benefit to patients with a smaller tumor burden?

The answer to this question obviously lies in controlled trials performed on patients with less advanced diseases.

References

1   Bansal, S. C.; Bansal, B. R.; Thomas, A. L.; Siegel, P. D.; Rhoads, J. E.; Cooper, D. R.; Terman, D. S.; Mark, R.: Ex vivo removal of serum IgG in a patient with colon carcinoma. Cancer 42: 1–18 (1978).
2   Browne O.; Bell, J.; Holland, P. D. J.; Thornes, R. D.: Plasmapheresis and immunostimulation. Lancet ii: 96 (1976).
3   Chiu, K. M.; Mortensen, R. F.; Osmand, A. P.; Gewurtz, H.: Interactions of α_1-acid glycoprotein with the immune system. I. Purification and effect upon lymphocyte responsiveness. Immunology 32: 997–1005 (1977).
4   Currie, G.: The role of circulating antigen as an inhibitor of tumour immunity in man. Br. J. Cancer 28: 153–161 (1973).
5   Guiliano, A. E.; Rangel, D.; Golub, S. H.; Holmes, E. C.; Morton, D. L.: Serum-mediated immunosuppression in lung cancer. Cancer 43: 917 (1979).
6   Heier, H. E.; Carpentier, N.; Lange, N.; Lamber, P. R.; Godal, T.: Circulating immune

complexes in patients with malignant lymphomas and solid tumors. Int. J. Cancer *20:* 887 (1977).

7 Hersey, P.; Isbister, J.; Edwards, A.; Murray, E.; Adams, E.; Biggs, J.; Milton, G. W.: Antibody-dependent cell-mediated cytotoxicity against melanoma cells induced by plasmapheresis. Lancet *i:* 825–828 (1976).

8 Hoffken, K.; Meredith, I. D.; Robins, A. R.; Baldwin, R. W.; Davies, C. J.; Blamey, R. W.: Circulating immune complexes in patients with breast cancer. Br. med. J. *ii:* 218 (1977).

9 Israel, L.; Edelstein, R.; Mannoni, P.; Radot, E.; Greenspan, E. M.: Plasmapheresis in patients with disseminated cancer: Clinical results and correlation with changes in serum protein. Cancer *40:* 3146–3154 (1977).

10 Israel, L.; Edelstein, R.: In vivo and in vitro studies on non-specific blocking factors of host origin in cancer patients: Role of plasma exchange as an immunotherapeutic modality. Israel J. med. Scis *14:* 105–130 (1978).

11 Israel, L.; Edelstein, R.; McDonald, J.; Weiss, J.; Schein, P.: Immunological and plasma protein changes in cancer patients following a single plasmapheresis. Biomed. Eng. *28:* 292 (1978).

12 Israel, L.; Edelstein, R.; Samak, R.; Baudelot, J.; Breau, J. L.; Mannoni, P.; Radot, E.: Clinical results of multiple plasmapheresis in patients with advanced cancer. In: Rosenfeld, Serrou (eds.), Immune Complexes and Plasma Exchanges in Cancer Patients, pp. 309–327 (Elsevier/North-Holland, Amsterdam 1981).

13 Israel, L.; Samak, R.; Edelstein, R.; Bogucki, D.; Breau, J. L.: Mise en évidence du rôle immunodépresseur des protéines de l'inflammation. Leur rôle physiopathologique chez les cancéreux. Annls Méd. int. *132:* 26–29 (1981).

14 Israel, L.; Samak, R.; Edelstein, R.; Bogucki, D.; Samak, M.: Immune-inhibiting properties of some acute-phase proteins – a possible mechanism of 'immune escape' in cancer. In: Rosenfeld, Serrou (eds.), New trends in human immunology and cancer immunotherapy, pp. 533–546 (Doin-Sanders, Paris 1980).

15 Izumi, T.; Nagai, S.; Suginoshita, T.: Serum immunosuppression test as a new tool for immunodiagnosis of lung cancer. Cancer Res. *40:* 444–447 (1980).

16 Mannick, J. A.; Contantian, M.; Pardridge, D.; Saporoschetz, I.; Badger, A.: Improvement of phytohemagglutinin responsiveness of lymphocytes from cancer patients after washing in vitro. Cancer Res. *37:* 3066–3070 (1977).

17 Rangel, D. M.; Golub, S. H.; Morton, D. L.: Demonstration of lymphocyte blastogenesis-inhibiting factors in sera of melanoma patients. Surgery *82:* 244 (1977).

18 Samak, R.; Israel, L.; Edelstein, R.: Influence of tumor burden, tumor removal, immune stimulation plasmapheresis on monocyte mobilization in cancer patients. In: Escobar, Friedman (eds.), Macrophages and lymphocytes, part B, pp. 411–423 (Plenum Publishing Corporation, New York 1980).

19 Sample, N. F.; Gertner, H. R.; Chretien, P. B.: Inhibition of phytohemagglutinin-induced in vitro lymphocyte transformation by serum from patients with carcinomata. J. natn. Cancer Inst. *42:* 1291 (1971).

20 Silk, M.: Effect of plasma from patients with carcinoma on in vitro lymphocyte transformation. Cancer *20:* 2088–2089 (1967).

21 Sjögren, H. O.; Hellström, I.; Bansal, S. C.; Hellström, K. E.: Suggestive evidence that the 'blocking antibodies' of tumor-bearing individuals may be antigen-antibody complexes. Proc. natn. Acad. Sci. USA *68:* 1372–1375 (1971).

22 Terman, D. S.; Yamamoto, T.; Mattioli, M.; Cook, G.; Tillquist, R.; Henry, J.; Poster, R.; Daskal, Y.: Extensive necrosis of spontaneaous canine mammary adenocarcinoma after extracorporeal perfusion over Staphylococcus aureus Cowan I. J. Immun. *124:* 795–805 (1980).

23 Wang, B. S.; Badger, A. M.; Nimber, R. R.; Cooperband, S. R.; Schmid, K.; Mannick, J. A.: Suppression of tumor-specific cell-mediated cytotoxicity by immunoregulatory alpha-globulin and by immunoregulatory alphaglobulin-like peptides from cancer patients. Cancer. Res. *37:* 3022 (1977).

Lucien Israel, MD, Immunotherapy Unit, Hôpital Avicenne, University Paris XIII, F-93000 Bobigny

Problems of Plasma-Exchange Solutions, Gamma-Globulin Substitution, and Tumor Enhancement in Plasmapheresis of Tumor Patients

J.-H. Beyer[1], M. Klee, U. Kaboth, A. Kehl, H. Köstering, G. Krieger, G. A. Nagel

Medizin. Univ.-Klinik, Abt. Hämatologie/Onkologie, Göttingen, FRG

Plasmapheresis has become a standard procedure for the treatment of various diseases such as hyperviscosity syndrome and diseases with auto-immune antibodies. More recently it has been employed as an experimental method for treating multiple forms of malignant diseases (table I).

The technical aspects of plasmapheresis as well as the possibilities of the specific removal of those substances, thought to be responsible for the disease, have been dealt with in the first part of this book. The manner in which we perform plasmapheresis has been reported by *Klee* in chapter IV. Those exchange solutions most frequently used are fresh-frozen plasma (FFP), plasma-protein fractions (PPF) in Ringer solution (5.7), and a 5% human albumin-saline (HA) solution (3.4).

FFP has the advantage of containing all normal components of human plasma that are necessary for a successful and safe exchange, for example the clotting factors. However, the following disadvantages are associated with FFP: an increased risk of hepatitis; in the case of rare blood groups, plasma is not usually available in sufficient quantity (10–15 l are required per exchange); an increased number of incompatibility reactions occur, caused by the presence of proteins foreign to the patient and the stabilizing solutions (calcium antagonists) in the plasma; metabolic studies on individual plasma components that could be involved in tumor growth are made more difficult since FFP may also contain these components.

[1] with a grant from the Fazit-Foundation.

Table I. Indications for plasma exchange

(1) Certain indications
 – Hyperviscosity syndromes
 – Thyrotoxic crisis
 – Severe myasthenia gravis
 – RH-incompatibility
 – Intoxications, e.g. Paraquad® intoxication

(2) Probable indications
 – Systemic lupus erythematosus
 – Immune complex nephritis
 – Goodpasture's syndrome
 – Wegener's granulomatosis
 – Raynaud's syndrome and other forms of vasculitis
 – Idiopathic thrombocytopenic purpura

(3) Possible indications
 – Hyperthyroidism
 – Resistance to insulin due to autoantibodies
 – Autoimmune hemolytic anemia
 – Pemphigus vulgaris

(4) Experimental indications
 – Malignant diseases
 – Immune deficiencies on the basis of serological changes
 – Autoimmune liver diseases (lupoid hepatitis; primary biliary cirrhosis)

The 5% human albumin-saline solution has the advantage that it can be used independent of the patient's blood group, and it is also always available. In addition, using this standardized solution containing a single protein, namely the albumin, allows for the above mentioned metabolic investigations of substances that can possibly influence tumor growth. The major disadvantage of this solution, and also of PPF, is its lack of clotting factors. Thus in exchanging large volumes of plasma, the danger is that an impoverishment of these factors may occur with the risk of bleedings. We have investigated the coagulating properties in 12 normal donors on repeated plasmapheresis. Every second day 100% of the calculated plasma volume of each donor was exchanged with HA up to five times. No increased bleeding risk was observed during these procedures. Then we felt secure in applying this method to 15 cancer patients. Caution is certainly justified since these patients may have a labile clotting system which can be further deranged by the plasma exchange in the sense of hypercoagulability or increased bleeding.

The data with regard to these problems are presented by *Köstering* in chapter IV. Another disadvantage is the possible occurrence of rare anaphylactic reactions [18].

We have now performed a total of 24 plasmapheresis-periods involving 91 individual plasmaphereses on these 15 cancer patients. A further 120 plasmaphereses have been carried out on patients with other symptoms. The side effects due to this plasma-exchange therapy are extremely small. Patients felt occasionally unwell after exchange with HA. Minor reactions were observed against FFP such as an itching of the skin, isolated exanthemas, and a tingling sensation around the mouth, in the toes and fingers. A drop in blood pressure occurred in only four plasmaphereses. We did not see any of the serious side reactions reported by *Aufeuvre* in chapter I. This is perhaps due to the fact that we have as yet performed only a relatively small number (210) of plasmaphereses.

In 1958 *Kaliss* [14] defined immunological enhancement as 'the successful establishment of a tumor homograft and its progressive growth (usually to death of the host) as a consequence of the tumor's contact with specific antiserum in the host'. This was later altered to 'the successful establishment or prolonged survival (conversely the delayed rejection) of an allogenic graft' [1, 15, 16, 17].

The mechanisms of tumor enhancement are multiform and extremely complex. As yet no clear picture has emerged from the numerous studies that have been made. The most important mechanisms can be considered to be the afferent, efferent, and central enhancement in which the following are involved; antigens, antibodies, antigen-antibody complexes, immunoglobulins, the host, blocking and deblocking serum factors, the various forms of immunity-mediated T-cells, suppressor T-cells, K-cells, natural K-cells, and macrophages.

It has also been suggested that unspecific serum-blocking factors such as acute-phase proteins can affect tumor enhancement. The following are under discussion: α1-antitrypsin, α2-macroglobulin, coeruloplasmin, haptoglobin, and orosomucoid, as well as the α1-, α2-, and γ-globulins [12, 13].

Low molecular-weight substances such as opsonines, lymphokines, the α2-pregnancy- associated antigen (α2-PAG), and prostaglandin E2 may also be immunosuppressive factors that play a role in the cell interaction of tumor enhancement.

The results of our studies on the acute-phase proteins have been differentiated according to the three different forms of plasmapheresis employed: (1) exchange with HA, (2) exchange with HA followed by

additions of 15–20 g Intraglobin®, Biotest, Frankfurt (a preparation containing intact immunoglobulins) after the last plasmapheresis, (3)
exchange with FFP.

A reduction in the levels of α1-antitrypsin was observed after all
forms of plasmapheresis but the original level was reattained the following
day. In the subsequent observation period no further major increase in
these values occurred (fig. 1).

Levels of α2-macroglobulin were reduced by 25–50% after all three
forms of plasmapheresis. On completion of the series of plasmaphereses
these values recovered only very slowly over an observation period of 5
days, and did not reach their original levels.

Little effect was observed on coeruloplasmin on exchange with FFP
whereas a reduction of 50% was found when using HA. The original
values were reattained within 4–5 days irrespective as to whether gammaglobulin had been added or not.

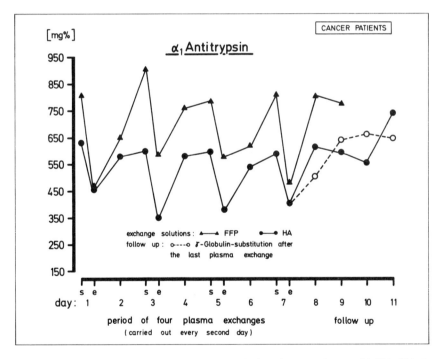

Fig. 1. Behavior of α1-antitrypsin during and after plasma exchange with HA, HA +
γ-globulin, and FFP.

α2-globulin was suppressed by all three forms of plasmapheresis, but the greatest effect was observed with HA. The values then recovered within 3–4 days.

No essential change occurred in transferrin concentrations after exchange with FFP. After exchange with HA, the values reduced by 50 % and recovered after 4–5 days. However, when gammaglobulin was added at the end of the plasmapheresis, no such recovery was observed after 5 days and the levels remained 50 % below the original values.

Thus transferrin proved to be the exception among the acute-phase proteins. Under the different forms of plasmapheresis its levels could be suppressed for the period of observation by adding gammaglobulin (fig. 2). An explanation for this phenomenon cannot as yet be proposed. The remaining acute-phase proteins did not differ essentially from one another.

In contrast to the clinical picture, no differences were observed in the measured levels of the acute-phase proteins whether the therapy was successful or not. Even when a progression of the tumor occurred under

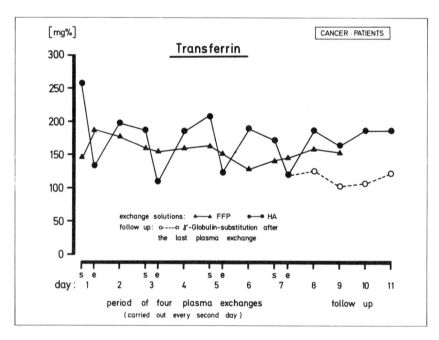

Fig. 2. Behavior of transferrin during and after plasma exchange with HA, HA + γ-globulin, and FFP.

plasmapheresis followed by the previously unsuccessful chemotherapy, a reduction in the acute-phase proteins was observed without affecting their immunosuppressive activities. A similar reduction in the acute-phase proteins was also observed in those patients who profitted from the above therapy.

The immune complexes are considered as belonging to specific blocking factors. They consist of antigen-antibody complexes which can develop, for example through the leaching of specific antigens from the tumor-cell surface, soluble immune complexes with specific antibodies. These can often bind lymphocytes and thus block the lymphocyte-mediated immune responses. This effect can be relieved by washing the lymphocytes or by the absence of the antigen in vitro. The renewed lymphocytes are again able to demonstrate their cytotoxic effect on target tumor cells. This process, therefore, appears to be reversible.

Various investigations have shown that the immune complexes possess both free antigen and antibody sites, which would explain the specificity of the blocking process.

Sjögren et al. [22, 23] showed that the blocking immune complexes, when separated from the serum of tumor-bearing mice through ultrafiltration at pH 3.1, disintegrate into two components neither of which demonstrate any blocking effects on their own. Only after remixing the two components, could any effect be observed. Similar results have been obtained by *Baldwin* [2] although in certain cases lymphocyte-mediated cytotoxicity was blocked by the antigen alone. However, this latter blocking effect need not necessarily have immunological specificity.

The blocking factors function by occupying lymphocyte receptors with antigen. The antibody component is possibly required for transporting the antigen to the lymphocyte or for fixing the antigen to the receptor. It appears to be especially necessary at low-antigen concentrations. A simplified explanation for deblocking could then be imagined if antibodies bind the antigen sites of the blocking complexes, or if they bind the antigen molecules in such a way that the antigen is no longer available to interact with the lymphocytes.

In this way cytotoxic activity of the lymphocytes would be protected. If the circulating immune complexes really represent blocking factors, then the detachment of antigen containing ligands from growing tumor cells would be of utmost importance and could lead to the suppression of the immunological control system. Tumor antigens could stimulate immunocompetent cells to produce antibodies. Through continuous production of antigen by the growing tumor, blocking immune complexes could then develop. It is even possible that the antibody-mediated cytotoxicity of lymphocytes is blocked when the antibody is bound by free antigen to form an immune complex.

In this manner the circulating immune complexes influence the tumor cells and the immunocompetent lymphocytes. All groups of lymphocytes such as the B- and T-cells, as well as the sub-group of T-cells such as the suppressor T-cells, killer-cells, and the macrophages are probably subject to this influence.

In addition to the previously described autoimmune diseases, circulating immunecomplexes have now been found in various tumor types: breast cancer, cancer of the colon, melanoma, osteogenic sarcoma, Hodgkin- and Non-Hodgkin-lymphoma, and leukemia. In some cases it was possible to make a prognosis of the disease based on the amount of measured immune complexes and their development. Unfortunately, in many cases, circulating immune complexes are not detectable, neither in the early nor late stages of the disease. When immune complexes are detected in connection with a malignancy, they can be eliminated by splenectomy, removal of the tumor, immunosuppressive therapy, ductus thoracicus drainage, or plasmapheresis [6, 10, 11].

In our 15 patients with malignant tumors who had several plasmapheresis treatments, we have twice detected highly elevated levels of immune complexes, in one case through the C_{1q}-binding method of Nydegger [19] and once with the laser-nephelometric method of Helmke [9].

The first patient was a 62-year-old man with a squamous cell carcinoma of the bronchus in which very high levels of immune complexes were measured. In the course of plasmapheresis therapy they were markedly reduced, but on cessation of the therapy they regained their original values within 3 weeks (fig. 3). In the other patient, a 48-year-old man with a highly malignant Non-Hodgkin-lymphoma, a rebound phenomenon of the originally normal values of the immune complexes was observed before the second plasmapheresis. However, the levels returned to normal during the course of treatment, although clinically a progression of the disease was observed during therapy (fig. 4). Only when the previously unsuccessful chemotherapy was again applied after the plasmapheresis therapy, a regression of the tumor was observed for about three weeks.

In order to avoid this rebound phenomenon, which has also been described by other authors, we conclude that repeated plasmapheresis is

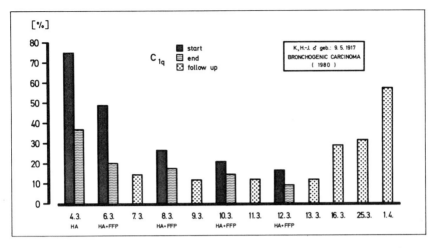

Fig. 3. Behavior of the circulating immune complexes during and after plasma exchange (measured by the C_{1q}-binding assay) in a patient with bronchogenic carcinoma.

necessary to prevent tumor enhancement due to excessive immune complex formation.

It should be theoretically possible to remove circulating immunecomplexes and other inhibitory substances through exchange therapy and thus achieve a better immunological basis with which the host is able to combat his disease. In all probability such an exchange therapy must be applied at a much earlier stage rather than at the end of all other forms of effective therapy, if it should be successful in improving the immunological situation of the patient. It is also plausible that an enhancement and progression of the tumor may occur due to the removal of factors that hinder its growth. Such phenomena are known from animal experiments, but have yet only been discussed in humans. In our 15 patients we have not been able to confirm any tumor enhancement. After completion of the plasmapheresis therapy, the patients were treated with the previously ineffective chemotherapy. In many cases they once again responded to this therapy, but only for a short period of 3–4 weeks. In the case of a malignant lymphoma the B-symptomatic and corticoid consumption was affected in a positive sense for a longer period of time.

According to our present experience, malignant lymphomas are most likely to respond to plasmapheresis with subsequent chemotherapy if all other forms of treatment have been fully tried. We have been able to establish that plasma exchange enriches the therapy of malignant tumors

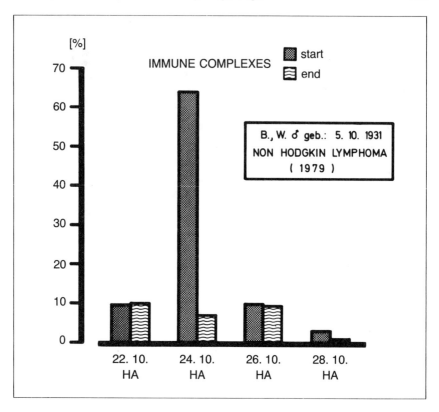

Fig. 4. Behavior of the circulating immune complexes during plasma exchange (measured by laser-nephelometry) in a patient with Non-Hodgkin-lymphoma.

in the case of patients who have become unresponsive to other forms of treatment.

Surface immunoglobulins can be detected on lymphocytes, macrophages, mast cells, granulocytes, and thrombocytes. B-cells and, according to recent results, T-cells can produce their own immunoglobulins. IgG, IgM, and IgD are to be found on the surface of B-cells whereas IgG and an altered IgM molecule are to be found on T-cells. These cells can also bind exogenously-formed immunoglobulins through their Fc-receptors. Surface-bound IgM is in most cases synthesized endogenously, as administration of gammaglobulins was intended to lead to a further reduction of circulating immune complexes, and, if possible, of specific antigen-antibody complexes. Further, the production of blocking factors should be hindered by the occupation of Fc-receptors on B-cells. Perhaps it is possible that in addition, a blockade of the T-cells can be achieved without blocking the tumor-destroying activity of the corresponding cells.

In these patients, who had plasma exchanges in this manner, no circulating immune complexes could be detected by the methods of *Nydegger, Helmke,* and *Theofilopoulos.* This question, therefore, remains open.

Surprisingly, in plasma exchanges with Intraglobulin® the initial rise in the gammaglobulin values over the first two days was followed by a marked decrease after the third day, whereas after exchange with FFP and HA alone a gradual increase or a constant behavior was observed (fig. 5). The same behavior was detected at IgG levels.

Due to their rapid metabolism IgA and IgM are unaffected by exchange with either HA or FFP, and their values remained constant during plasmapheresis therapy. However, after gammaglobulin substitu-

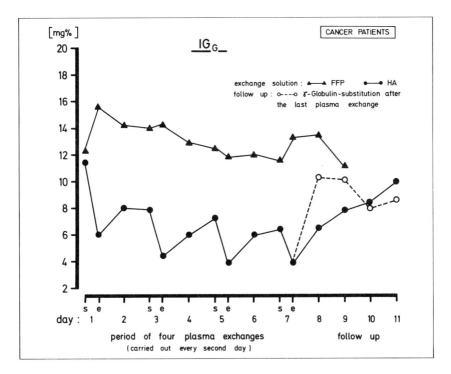

Fig. 5. Behavior of IgG during and after plasma exchange with HA, HA + γ-globulin, and FFP.

tion the IgA values were reduced by 50%, and the levels were maintained over the next five days. Similar observations were also made with IgM whose values were reduced up to 50% (figs. 6 and 7).

From these data we can conclude that the production of immuno-globulins is suppressed by the administration of 15–20 g of Intraglobulin® after the last plasmapheresis and that this suppression lasts at least five days. This is in contrast to exchanges with FFP and HA alone in which a clear increase in the suppressed levels occurred after the end of the plas-mapheresis. Whether gammaglobulin substitution simply causes a reduc-tion in the production of unspecific gammaglobulins or whether it also causes a suppression of specific immunoglobulins (e.g. specific antibodies, in which the new production of antigen-antibody complexes is hindered), cannot be distinguished at the moment. However, it appears to influence the B-cell function of immunoglobulin production. The clinical course of the disease in our patients also showed a temporary but distinct improve-ment when using this form of plasmapheresis.

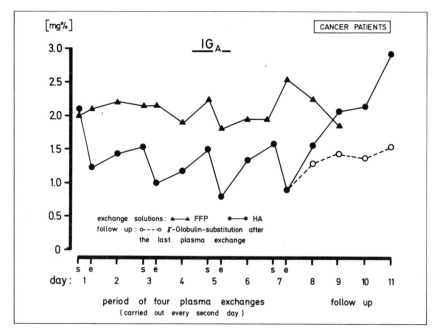

Fig. 6. Behavior of IgA during and after plasma exchange with HA, HA + γ-globulin, and FFP.

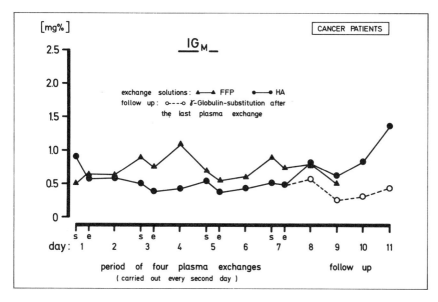

Fig. 7. Behavior of IgM during and after plasma exchange with HA, HA + γ-globulin, and FFP.

Many questions remain to be answered. Can the immunological state of tumor patients be further improved by earlier use of plasmapheresis compared to its present application? Can subsequent chemotherapy improve the clinical course of the disease? Is a single plasma exchange of 10–15 1 better than sequential plasmaphereses of 3 1 every second day? Does substitution with HA really offer advantages over exchange with FFP? Is a higher gammaglobulin substitution better than the present dosage of 10–15 g and should it be employed after every plasmapheresis and not just during the last one of a series?

The list of questions can easily be extended.

References

1   Alexander, P.: In: Anderson (ed.), The biology and surgery of tissue transplantation (Davis, Philadelphia 1970).
2   Baldwin, R. W.; Price, M. R.; Robin, R. A.: Blocking of lymphocyte-mediated cytotoxicity for rat hepatoma cells by tumor-specific antigen-antibody complexes. Nature *238:* 185 (1972).
3   Beyer, J.-H.; Klee, M.; Bartsch, H.-H.; Borghardt, J.; Brockmeyer, J.; Kaboth, U.;

Köstering, H.; Bolling, R.; Nagel, G. A.: First experiment with plasmapheresis in patients with neoplastic diseases. 15th German Cancer Congress, Munich, March 11–15, 1980.

4 Beyer, J.-H.; Klee, M.; Kehl, A.; Krieger, G.; Bartsch, H.-H.; Borghardt, J.; Brockmeyer, J.; Kaboth, U.; Köstering, H.; Nagel, G. A.: Erste klinische Erfahrungen mit dem großvolumigen Plasmaaustausch bei Patienten mit malignen Erkrankungen. Schw. med. Wschr. *110:* 1447–1449 (1980).

5 Farrales, F. B.; Summers, T.; Belcher, C.; Bayer, W. L.: Plasma exchange with plasma protein fraction and lactated Ringer's solution using the continous flow cell separator. Infusionstherapie *2:* 273–277 (1975).

6 Ferrer, J. F.; Mihich, E.: Effect of splenectomy in the regression of transplantable tumors. Cancer Res. *28:* 1116 (1968).

7 Flaum, M. A.; Cuneo, R. A.; Appelbaum, F. R.; Deisseroth, A. B.; King-Engel, W.; Gralunick, H. R.: The hemostatic of plasma-exchange transfusion. Blood (54) *3:* 694–702 (1979).

8 Gally, J. A.; Edelman, G. M.: The genetic control of immunoglobulin synthesis. Ann. Rev. Med. *6:* 1–46 (1972).

9 Helmke, K.; Sodomann, C. P.; Teuber, I.; Federlin, K.: Nachweis zirkulierender Immunkomplexe mit der Laser-Nephelometrie. Immunität und Infektion *6:* 173–179 (1978).

10 Heppner, G. H.: Blocking antibodies and enhancement. Ser. Haematol. *5:* 41 (1972).

11 Heppner, G. H.; Griswold, D. E.; Di Lorenzo, J. et al.: Selective immunosuppression by drugs in balanced immune responses. Fed. Proc. *33:* 1882 (1974).

12 Israel, L.; Edelstein, R.; Mannoni, P.; Radot, E.; Greenspan, E. M.: Plasmapheresis in patients with disseminated cancer: Clinical results and correlation with changes in serum protein. The concept of 'non-specific blocking factors'. Cancer *40:* 3146–3154 (1977).

13 Israel, L.; Edelstein, R.: In vivo and in vitro studies on nonspecific blocking factors of host origin in cancer patients. Role of plasma exchange as an immunotherapeutic modality. J. Med. Soc. *14:* 105–130 (1978).

14 Kaliss, N.: Immunological enhancement of tumor homografts in mice; a review. Cancer Res. *18:* 992–1003 (1958).

15 Kaliss, N.: The elements of immunological enhancement: A consideration of mechanism. Ann. N.Y. Acad. Sci. *101:* 64–69 (1962).

16 Kaliss, N.: Immunological enhancement. In: Najarian, Simmons (eds.), Transplantation, p. 195 (Lea and Febiger, Philadelphia 1972).

17 McKhann, C. F.: Immunologic enhancement. In: Najarian, Simmons (eds.), Transplantation, p. 305 (Lea and Febiger, Philadelphia 1972).

18 McMillin, R. D.; Hood, T. R.; Griffen, W. O. jr.: Systemic anaphylaxis secondary to the use of 5 per cent plasma protein fractions. Amer. J. Surg. *135:* 706–707 (1978).

19 Nydegger, U. E.; Lambert, P. H.; Gerber, H.; Mischer, P. A.: Circulating immune complexes in the serum in systemic lupus erythematosus and in carriers of hepatitis B antigen. Quantitation by binding to radiolabeled C_{1q}. J. clin. Invest. *54:* 297–309 (1974).

20 Paraskevas, F.; Lees, S. T.; Orr, K. B.; Israels, L. G.: A receptor for Fc on mouse B-lymphocytes. J. Immunol. *108:* 1319–1327 (1972).

21 Schwenk, H. U.; Baenkler, H. W.: Effect of gammaglobulin injection on circulating immune complexes in various diseases. Europ. J. Pediatr. *131:* 43–48 (1979).

22 Sjögren, H. O.; Hellström, I.; Bansal, S. C.; Hellström, K. E.: Suggestive evidence that the blocking antibodies of tumor-bearing individuals may be antigen-antibody complexes. Proc. natn. Acad. Sci. (Wash.) *68:* 1375 (1971).

23   Sjögren, H. O.; Hellström, I.; Bansal, S. C.; Warner, G.; Hellström, K. E.: Elution of
     blocking factors from human tumors capable of abrogating tumor cell destruction by
     specifically immune lymphocytes. Int. J. Cancer 9: 274 (1972).

Dr, J.-H. Beyer, Abt. Hämatologie/Onkologie, Medizin. Universitäts-Klinik, Robert-Koch-
Str. 40, D-3400 Göttingen

Blood Coagulation Changes Induced by Repeated Plasmapheresis in 12 Normal Donors and 15 Patients with Malignomas

H. Köstering, J.-H. Beyer, M. Klee, U. Kasten, P. Schuff-Werner, G. A. Nagel

Medizin. Universitätsklinik, Abt. Hämatologie/Onkologie, Göttingen, FRG

Plasmapheresis has established itself in recent years in the treatment of patients with hyperviscosity syndromes, antibodies, or different malignant diseases [4, 5]. Previous investigations in hemodialysis patients [11] and patients undergoing operations aided by the heart-lung machine both with and without hemodilution [9, 10, 12] gave reason to fear that contact of the heparinized blood with the foreign membrane or the tube and pump system would also have effects on the coagulation system and thrombocytes of plasmapheresis patients. For these reasons, we initiated detailed coagulation studies at the start of plasmapheresis treatment in both normal persons and patients, in order to monitor potentially harmful coagulation changes and to avoid them if possible. Furthermore, we were interested in the still unresolved problem of how many successive sessions of plasmapheresis can be applied and how often coagulation factors can be withdrawn from the patient without his requiring substitutions with human coagulation preparations [1, 5, 6]. The results of repeated plasmapheresis sessions in 12 normal persons and 15 patients with malignomas have now evaluated and this paper will briefly report on them.

Material and Methods

These studies were carried out in 12 normal persons, who showed normal values according to clinical and laboratory parameters, and 15 patients with different types of malignomas, of whom we will report in detail elsewhere.

Plasma exchange, was performed in a continuous-blood flow, using the IBM blood-cell separator 2997. Anticoagulation was achieved with doses of heparin. Initial dose of 5000 U heparin and continuous infusion of 1000 U/h were given. Blood-flow rate during the course of treatment was app. 40–60 ml/min. The plasma exchange volume was aimed at 4% body weight or 100% plasma volume of normal persons and patients. Plasma exchanges were performed consecutively on normal persons every 2nd day and up to 5 times [4, 5]. Patients with malignomas received plasmapheresis treatments every 2nd day also, but only 4 times consecutively.

The coagulation parameters of normal persons and patients were examined daily. After 60 min and at the end of every plasmapheresis treatment, and then continuously every 24 h, the normal persons' coagulation parameters were checked. This 60 min value was not checked in patients with malignomas. We performed this check in normal persons in order to register any changes during every course of treatment, thereby allowing an intervention of the treatment should it become necessary. Since this control check after 60 min did not result in any additional, important information and showed that normal persons had sufficient amounts of coagulants until the end of the treatment, we decided to omit this check in our patients. After 5 consecutive plasmapheresis treatments with a break of 1 day, we continued to check coagulation factors daily in order to register the recovery of those factors both in normal persons and patients. It proved useful to check the coagulation after 24, 48, 72, 96, and 336 h.

Plasmapheresis was also carried out every 2nd day in patients with malignomas, but usually only up to 4 times in succession. Four sessions of plasmapheresis have been presented in the evaluation of the data. In the 15 patients, a total of 21 courses of plasmapheresis were evaluated; the mean values and standard deviations are shown. After the 4th session of plasmapheresis had ended, the blood coagulation parameters were monitored continuously after 24, 48, 72, 96, 120, and 144 h. The data for the individual blood coagulation determinations has been compiled as mean values and standard deviations and is presented separately for both groups. Using commercial blood coagulation tests and coagulometers, photometers, and partigen plates [2, 3, 7, 8, 10], we carried out the following blood coagulation tests in the 12 normal persons and 21 plasmapheresis courses:

(1) PTT
(2) Thrombin time
(3) Quick's test
(4) Fibrinogen according to Schulz
(5) Fibrin-monomer complex (protamine-sulfate test)
(6) Factor XIII
(7) Factor VIII
(8) Factor V
(9) Factor II
(10) Thrombelastogram (r-time, k-time, maximum thrombus elasticity)
(11) Thrombocyte count
(12) Partigen immunodiffusion plates: antithrombin III, plasminogen, α_1-antitrypsin, α_2-macroglobulin, fibrinogen
(13) Fibrin platelets and heated fibrin plates
(14) Plasmin, antiplasmin, antithrombin III, heparin, and factor Xa were determined with chromogenic substrates.

The plasmapheresis procedures and our blood-coagulation investigations were the same for both groups. On the basis of our findings, we are convinced that we cannot dispense with anticoagulation with heparin for these patients. In order not to allow a further worsening of the possible activation of thrombocytes and the coagulation system due to contact of the heparinized blood with the foreign membrane, we did not inactivate the still circulating heparin at the end of plasmapheresis by administering protamine chloride.

In all cases plasmapheresis lasted until almost exactly 4% of the body weight had been exchanged. Altogether the duration of plasmapheresis amounted to approximately 120–150 min. The exchanged plasma was substituted by an equal volume of 5% human albumin solution in both normal persons and patients.

Results

(a) Investigations in 12 Normal Persons

The results of the thrombocyte counts are presented graphically in figure 1. In contrast to the initial values before commencement of plasmapheresis, there was an obvious and pronounced decline in thrombocytes after every treatment.

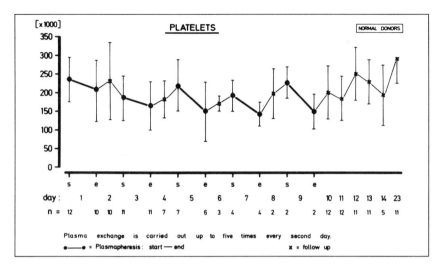

Fig. 1. Mean values and SEM of numbers of platelets in normal persons during and after repeated plasmapheresis.

It should be noted that between each plasmapheresis treatment, the thrombocyte count recovered. On completion of the plasmapheresis sessions the trombocyte count continued to rise and reached the baseline value already after 3 days. Figure 1 also indicates the presence of a considerable scatter in the thrombocyte counts. In no individual case, however, did the thrombocyte count fall to a dangerous level. The mean values also demonstrate that no risk can be expected from the effect of plasmapheresis treatment on thrombocytes to normal persons.

The mean values presented in the results of the partial thromboplastin time (PTT) (see fig. 2) clearly show that, during plasmapheresis treatment, complete anticoagulation was attained in each case. In both the determinations of PTT and the thrombin time, our blood coagulation studies were basically ended after 5 min (300 s). However, it is striking that, despite continuous administration of 1000 U heparin/h during the treatment, the partial thromboplastin time indicated a tendency to normalization. Compared with basal values before the first plasmapheresis treatment, the global coagulation test was not lengthened. This is evident from the individual basal values of a renewed plasmapheresis session and also by the 24 h values. Moreover, the further course of the PTT was normal after conclusion of the 5th plasmapheresis session with normal donors. In no case was a curtailment or lengthening of the PTT observed.

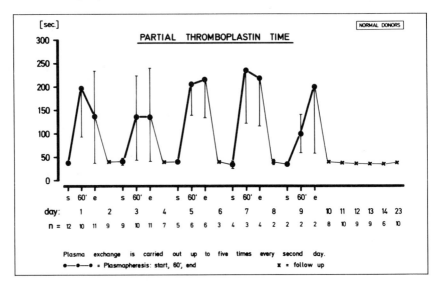

Fig. 2. Mean values and SEM of partial-thromboplastin-time (PTT) in normal donors.

For this reason, repeated plasmapheresis treatments seem to pose no danger of hypercoagulability or bleeding for normal persons.

The thrombin time behaved in a similar way (these values are not reported here). During the determination of the thrombin time, the greatest lengthening occurred after application of the initial dose; during continuous application of heparin (below 1000 U/h), a minor decline of the mean values occurred. At the end of plasmapheresis, there were no observations of a rebound phenomenon. The mean values, as well as an analysis of the individual data, indicated that a shortening of the thrombin time did not occur. This indication seems particularly important since occasionally, during long-term treatments with heparin, heparinase, the heparin-inactivating enzyme, is stimulated and produced in increased amounts, especially when heparin is administered in massive doses. According to the present results however, it would appear that there is no danger of this occurring if renal function is normal.

Likewise we dispense with the presentation of the antithrombin-III level, the heparin cofactor. According to the mean and individual values, the application of heparin resulted in an immediate decline in the antithrombin-III concentration; although it usually recovered its original level within 24 h. Nevertheless, during the course of consecutive treatments, the heparin cofactor declined, reaching its lowest value at the end of the 5th plasmapheresis session. However, already within 24 h of the final session, a normalizing trend was observed and, after 3 days, the anti-thrombin level in normal persons had again reached the original basal value observed before the 5 sessions of plasmapheresis.

Figure 3 clearly shows that the most pronounced decline during plas-mapheresis occurs in the fibrinogen level, which was determined with the aid of the heat-coagulation method according to Schulz. Fibrinogen con-centration fell from 330 mg% to 150 mg% during the 1st plasma exchange. During an interval of 48 h this level did not completely approach the basal value. In the course of 5 plasmapheresis sessions with normal persons, the mean value for fibrinogen fell continually. After the plasmapheresis sessions had been completed, it took 5 days for fibrinogen to reach the mean value observed prior to treatment. Although a clear decline was observed for the fibrinogen concentration, neither mean val-ues nor individual determinations indicated that a normal person would hemorrhage due to a low fibrin level.

Fibrinogen levels, determined immunologically by using partigen plates, behave similar to those determined by heat-coagulation method. Here, too, was a prompt decline of fibrinogen and a complete recovery did not occur within the next treatment-free 48 h. The results of this assay

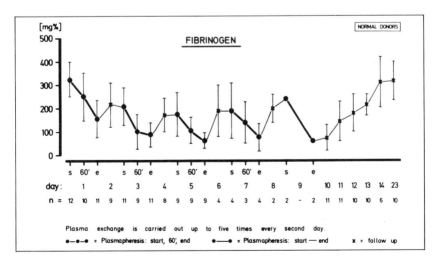

Fig. 3. Mean values and SEM of fibrinogen, determined by heat coagulation, in normal donors during and after treatment with plasmapheresis.

method also clearly showed that immunologically determined fibrinogen declines during plasmapheresis and only after all plasmapheresis treatments had ceased did a slow recovery take place.

Fluctuations, similar to those observed in the fibrinogen concentration, would also be expected in the maximal thrombus elasticity, as seen in the thrombelastogram. However, it is striking that the maximal elasticity was again recovered in almost all cases within 48 h. Only after the 4th and 5th sessions could this reduction not be compensated; here the value was clearly lower than the basal value before beginning the final plasmapheresis treatment. The maximal thrombus elasticity recovered within 5 days, as did the fibrinogen level. Here, too, we dispense with mean values and standard deviations due to lack of space.

The r-time in the thrombelastogram behaved similarly to the thrombin time. As was to be expected, the r- and k-times were much longer both during and at the end of plasmapheresis treatment. However, in no case was a longer or shorter r- or k-time observed after 24 or 48 h. The r- and k-times also recovered within 24 h of the last plasmapheresis treatment. From these results of the thrombelastogram, we can conclude that in no case was there danger of hypercoagulability or hemorrhaging to the normal donor, even after 5 plasmapheresis treatments.

The considerable decline in the mean values and standard deviations in normal persons already observed for the fibrinogen concentration was also apparent in the evaluation of factor XIII, the fibrin-stabilizing factor. Figure 4 shows the pronounced decline in factor XIII during plasmapheresis treatment. It is also evident from this figure that a further and continuing decline of the fibrin-stabilizing factor occurred during the treatment. The lowest value measured in a normal person was 25 % at the end of the 5th plasmapheresis session. Subsequently factor XIII recovered slowly, and 5 days after conclusion of the treatment it had reached its basal value again.

Special attention was paid during and after treatment to the behavior of the fibrin-monomer complexes in the blood of normal donors. Although there was considerable scatter in the individual values, at no time was there an elevation of this complex compared with the activation of the fibrinogen-sensitive protamine-sulfate test. Thus there was no indication of a continuing hypercoagulability in these patients after plasmapheresis was concluded. The individual results are not presented.

The largest fluctuations occurred in the results determined for factor VIII. During plasmapheresis there was a clear fall in activity, directly

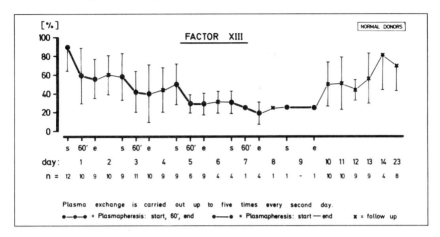

Fig. 4. Mean values and SEM of factor XIII in normal donors.

dependent on applied heparin. However, factor VIII always recovered completely within 24 h. Even after the last session, the factor VIII concentration remained within the normal range.

The blood coagulation investigations compiled to measure fibrinolytic activity clearly show (fig. 5) that plasminogen (the carri of fibrinolytic activity), whether determined by the chromogenic substrates or immunologically with partigen plates, declined markedly after every plasma exchange. However, it always recovered within 24 h. If plasminogen was activated to plasmin by streptokinase, a strong decline also appeared during plasmapheresis. Similar to plasmin, surprisingly, antiplasmin also declined. It is also noteworthy that, within 24 h after treatment, antiplasmin reached highly elevated values.

As was expected, the number of lysis plaques in the normal and heated fibrin plates rose during the plasmapheresis treatment. Thus a slightly increased fibrinolytic activity was observed during plasmapheresis. According to the mean values, the inhibitors of blood coagulation, α_2-macroglobulins (fig. 6), declined during plasmapheresis. This inhibitor did not completely recover within 24 h, thus the mean values before commencing another plasma exchange are clearly lower. Also after the final treatment, the mean values of this inhibitor increased only slowly. On the 5th day after the conclusion of treatment, α_2-macroglobulin did not completely reach the basal value. The determination of α_1-antitrypsin also indicated a decline during plasmapheresis; however, within 24 h this

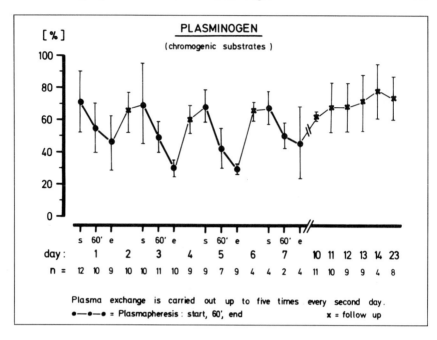

Fig. 5. Mean values and SEM of plasminogen levels, determined by chromogenic substrates in normal donors.

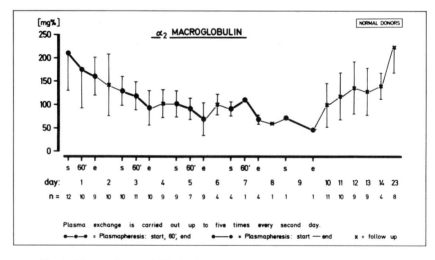

Fig. 6. Mean values and SEM of α_2-macroglobulin in normal donors, undergoing repeated plasmapheresis.

inhibitor had recovered its basal value. Similarly, after conclusion of treatment, the mean values were only slightly above the original basal values.

(b) Investigations in 15 Patients with Malignomas

The results from the blood coagulation studies in the 15 patients with malignomas, which were compiled from 21 evaluated plasmapheresis courses, were similar to the findings in the 12 normal persons. In this 2nd series, we dispensed with the 60-min value after commencing plasmapheresis, and the courses were carried out only for 4 days. Figure 7 depicts the results of the fibrinogen determination according to Schulz. As with the normal donors, here, too, was a clear decline. However, the basal values in these patients were considerably higher. After the treatment was completed, the fibrinogen level recovered but only very slowly. However, in no case did the reduction of fibrinogen concentration pose a threat to the patient.

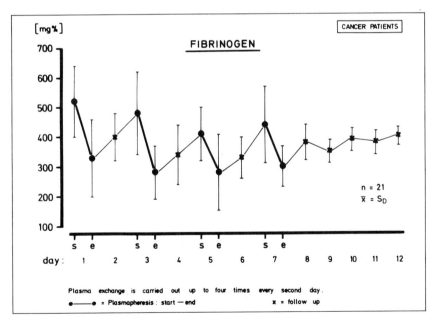

Fig. 7. Mean values and SEM of fibrinogen determinations in 15 patients with different malignomas during and after repeated (4 times) plasmapheresis.

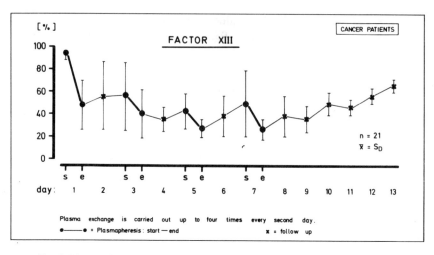

Fig. 8. Mean values and SEM of factor XIII in patients with malignomas.

Figure 8 presents the results for factor XIII, which were compiled from patients with carcinomas. The elevated mean values clearly show that there was also a pronounced decline in the fibrin-stabilizing factor. Likewise there was no complete recovery of the factor XIII-level during the 24–48 h between each treatment, therefore, the mean value continued to fall. The lowest value measured occurred at the end of the 4th plasmapheresis session and was 28 %. Within 6 days after the final session, the mean value recovered but did not completely reach the basal value.

Figure 9 depicts the behavior of the mean values in these patients for α_1-antitrypsin. During plasmapheresis there was a pronounced decline, but already after 24 h a normalizing tendency could be observed. Already 3 days after conclusion of the plasmapheresis treatment, the mean value was close to the α_1-antitrypsin level measured before each treatment.

The thrombocyte counts, PTT, thrombin time, the fibrin-monomer complexes, and factors VIII, V, and II reacted as in normal persons. No differences were found in the evaluations of the r- and k-times or the maximal thrombus elasticity in the thrombelastogram. Likewise the behavior of antithrombin III, plasminogen, plasmin, heated fibrin plates, and fibrin plates did not essentially differ from those in normal donors. Also a similar tendency as shown in the results of normal persons was seen in the mean values of α_2-macroglobulin, antiplasmin, and factor Xa, which showed only minimal differences.

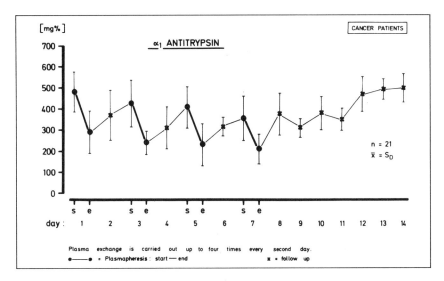

Fig. 9. Mean values and SEM of α₁-antitrypsin during and after plasmapheresis in 15 patients.

The coagulation factors were determined with chromogenic substrates using frozen plasma. For this reason, the determination of the heparin level was not reliable. Although the high-dose heparin therapy resulted in repeated, massive increases in heparin, the high levels yielded no information on reactions between plasma exchanges and after treatments. It is now known that heparin reacts very sensitively and yields dubious results when using frozen plasma, so that no predictions can be made on the basis of our investigations about the behavior of heparin after plasma exchanges.

For this reason, we will dispense with a detailed discussion and presentation of heparin.

Discussion

The findings presented here show that a clear decline in thrombocytes and fibrinogen occurs during plasmapheresis. Almost all coagulation factors decline; this is especially true for factor XIII. On the other hand, there is also a prompt activation of fibrinolytic activity and a fall in plasmin. This explains why the fibrin-monomer complexes, determined in our investigations with the protamine sulfate test, showed no increase during plasmapheresis, since they are obviously immediately lysed due to the activation of fibrinolysis. Thus the essential results from plasmapheresis treatment correspond to those obtained with the heart-lung machine [9, 10, 12] and hemodialysis [11]. Unfortunately a determination of the fibrin degradation products (antithrombin VI) was not within the scope of this investigation. However, it can be assumed that these fibrin degradation products will show an increase.

Factor XIII surprisingly declined to an especially pronounced extent. According to the results, the synthesis rate in this fibrin-stabilizing factor, which has a half-life of 82–96 h, seems to be clearly less than that of the other coagulation factors. The decline of this factor continually increased. Likewise the recovery time for factor XIII was the slowest. Thus, factor XIII may possibly be a limiting factor for long-term plasmapheresis treatments.

It could not be determined whether the contact of the heparinized blood with the pump-tube system and the foreign membrane played a role in considerably intensifying the decline in the coagulation factors. However, it can be assumed that a major portion of the thrombocytes and fibrinogen were depleted on these foreign membranes. In no case did the decline and elimination of the coagulation factors become so extensive as to be life-threatening, as the findings showed in long-term investigations in normal persons and patients with malignomas.

References

1 Bayer, W. L.; Farrales, F. B.; Summers, T.; Belcher, C.: Coagulation studies after plasma exchange with plasma protein fraction and lactated Ringer's solution. In Goldman and Lowenthal (eds), Leucocytoses: Separation, Collection and Transfusion, pp. 551–560 (Academic Press, London, New York, San Francisco 1975).

2 Behring-Werke: Laboratoriumsblätter für medizinische Diagnostik Nr. 4 (Farbwerke Hoechst, Frankfurt 1974).

3 Behring-Werke: Partigen-Immundiffusionsplatten (Farbwerke Hoechst, Frankfurt 1974).

4 Beyer, J. H.; Klee, M.; Bartsch, H.-H.; Borghardt, J.; Brockmeyer, J.; Kaboth, U.; Köstering, H.; Bolling, R.; Nagel, G. A.: First experiences with plasmapheresis in patients with neoplastic diseases. 15. German Cancer Congress (Munich, March 1980).

5 Beyer, H. J.; Klee, M.; Köstering, H.; Nagel, G. A.: Coagulation studies before, during, and after repeated plasma exchanges with a 5% human albumin/saline solution in normal donors. In: Siebert (ed.), International Symposium in Cologne, June 1980 (Schattauer Verlag, Stuttgart, 1980).

6 Farrales, F. B.; Summers, T.; Belcher, C.; Bayer, W. L.: Plasma exchanges with plasma protein fraction and lactated Ringer's solution using the continuous-flow cell separator. Infusionstherapie 2: 273–277 (1975).

7 Hartert, H.: Thrombelastography. In: Bang, Keller, Deutsch, and Mammen (eds.) Thrombosis and bleeding disorders, pp. 70–76 (Thieme, Stuttgart 1971).

8 Hoffmann-La Roche: Einführung in die Methodik der Blutgerinnungsbestimmungen (Hoffmann-La Roche, Grenzach 1969).

9 Köstering, H.: Veränderung der Blutgerinnung bei Hämodilution. 7. Internationale Fortbildungs- und Arbeitstagung des Verbandes der Kardiotechniker Deutschlands e. V. (Göttingen, Mai 1978).

10 Köstering, H.: Die Thromboembolien (Schattauer Verlag, Stuttgart–New York 1981).

11 Köstering, H.; Mietzsch, G.; Tönnis, H. J.; Quellhorst, E.; Scheler, F.: Blutungsbereitschaft unter der Hämodialyse durch intermembranösen Verbrauch von Thrombozyten und Gerinnungsfaktoren. Med. Welt 23: 1749–1752 (1972).

12 Köstering, H.; Kirchhoff, P. G.; Völker, P.; Warmann, E.; Koncz, J.: Blutgerinnungsveränderungen während und nach Anwendung der Herz-Lungen-Maschine und deren medikamentöse Beeinflussung. Z. Thorax vaskul. Chir. 21: 534–543 (1973).

13 Lipinsky, B.; Worowski, K.: Detection of soluble fibrin monomere complexes by means of protamine-sulfate-test. Thromb. Diath. haemorrh. 20: 44–49 (1968).

Prof. Dr. H. Köstering, Medizin. Universitätsklinik, Abt. Hämatologie/Onkologie, Robert-Koch-Str. 40, D-3400 Göttingen

Plasma Exchange
in a Case of Autoimmune Hemolytic Anemia
with Temporary Evan's Syndrome

H. Mönch[1], R. Lynen[2], J.-H. Beyer[1], C. Mueller-Eckhardt[3]

[1] Zentrum für Innere Medizin, Göttingen, FRG
[2] Blutspendezentrale der Universität Göttingen, FRG
[3] Institut für klinische Immunologie und Transfusionsmedizin des Klinikums der Justus-Liebig-Universität Gießen, FRG

Case Study

In April 1980 a 72-year-old female patient was presented at the hospital with general pallor, dizziness, vomiting, and jaundice. At the time of admission, the patient showed the following clinical signs of hemolysis: erythrocyte count of 1.96 million/mm^3, hemoglobin of 7.9 g%, bilirubin = 4.0 g%, LDH of 942 U/l, and 541‰ reticulocytes. Haptoglobin could not be measured. The thrombocyte count amounted to 285 000/mm^3, and bone-marrow histology showed a high degree of hyperplasia of the erythropoesis. After ruling out the possibility of a systemic disease, the detection of IgG antibodies and complement (C_3d) fixed in the erythrocytes and an auto-D antibody of the IgM type led to a diagnosis of an autoimmune hemolytic anemia. Following a subsequent decline in thrombocytes, that was triggered by thrombocytic antibodies, the diagnosis was changed to Evan's syndrome, the combination of an autoimmune hemolytic anemia and thrombocytopenia [1, 2].

Methods

The blood group, Rh-factor, and presence of erythrocytic antibodies were determined in a routine serologic examination. For this examination we used polyvalent anti-human globulin sera supplied by Ortho Diagnostics and the Behringwerke (Marburg), monospecific agglutinating Coombs' sera of anti-IgM, anti-IgG, anti-IgA, and anti-C_3d specificities provided by the companies Biotest (Frankfurt/Main) and Merz & Dade (Munich). Experiments were carried out to ascertain the specificity of auto-antibodies by using erythrocyte eluates and by gel-chromatographic fractionation of the patient's citrate plasma (Biogel A5m).

The hemolytically effective serum complement was determined according to a modification of the method of *Kabat and Mayer* [4] by establishing the CH_{50} units. Sensitized sheep erythrocytes (EA) were incubated for 60 min at 37°C with increasing amounts of human serum diluted 1:100 (0.1 ml × 10^8 EA/ml up to 0.3 ml serum at 1:100, veronal buffer to 1 ml). Subsequently, the extent of hemolysis was photometrically measured (412 nm) by determining the hemoglobin in the supernatant. After establishing the number of CH_{50} units, the contents of single samples were given in percentages with reference to a serum pool of 15 healthy blood donors. The norm range was established to be 100% ± 20% ($\bar{x}$ ± 2 SD, n = 15).

Thrombocytic antibodies were determined by the radioimmune antiglobulin test (for details on this method see [3]).

Results

The treatment was initiated with 150 mg Decortin. Four weeks after onset of therapy, the thrombocyte count fell to 12000/mm³. The radioimmune antiglobulin test [3] yielded proof of cell-fixed thrombocytic antibodies.

While continuing the Decortin therapy, the patient also received Imurek. Moreover, plasmapheresis was considered necessary and was carried out at first 5 times every 2nd day. Each exchange was performed with 4–5 l human albumin.

After the 5th session, plasma exchange had to be discontinued because of the appearance of several lung emboli. When, at a later time, new lung emboli developed in the patient after the 6th session of plasma exchange, immunosuppression with Imurek was continued and the administration of Decortin was gradually withdrawn. A rise in thrombocytes took place 14 days after the plasma-exchange therapy, and 4 weeks later they were in the norm range and thrombocytic antibodies could no longer be detected (fig. 1).

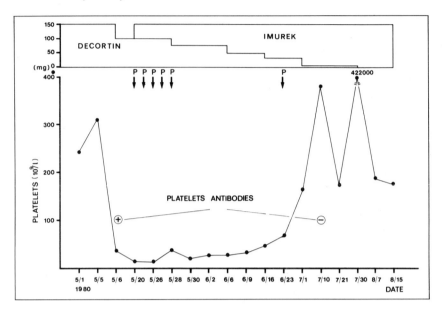

Fig. 1. Course of the thrombocyte values during administration of Decortin and Imurek and plasma-exchange therapy at the time of hospitalization from May to August 1980.

At no time were free erythrocytic antibodies detected in the patient's serum. To objectively evaluate the success of plasma-exchange therapy, the erythrocytic antibodies were titrated in a direct anti-human globulin test against a polyvalent anti-human globulin serum. Although the antibody load was reduced during the plasma-exchange therapy, the baseline value was reached again only 1 week after the last exchange session. Approximately 10 days after the 5th plasma exchange session, there was a clear rise in the reticulocyte values and a slight increase in the Hb value. However, during this same period, there was no further decline in the LDH value. Bilirubin and haptaglobin showed no appreciable improvement (fig. 2).

Since complement was involved in the hemolytic process, its level was followed during plasmapheresis. Figure 3 shows the individual plasma-exchange sessions according to the complement level which is measured in CH_{50} units [4]. These units are designated as percentages of the norm (see fig. 3). Each single plasma-exchange session considerably lowers the complement level, of which the baseline value is in the lower norm range. Two days later a renewed increase to 85% of the baseline value was measured.

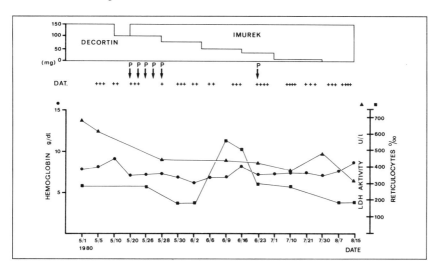

Fig. 2. Clinical course of the patient and course of the erythrocytic antibodies during hospitalization from May to August 1980.

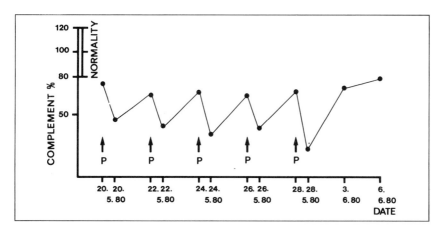

Fig. 3. Complement level during plasma-exchange therapy.

The effect of repeated plasma exchanges is not additive. Thus, only a temporary lowering of the complement level could be achieved with plasma exchange, but no long-term rise into the norm range.

Table I. Lab test data for the patient L. L. at the time of hospitalization and release

		Admission	Dismissal
Erythrocytes	$(10^{12}/l)$	1,96	2,54
Hemoglobin	(g/dl)	7,9	8,5
Platelets	$(10^9/l)$	285	187
Bilirubin	(mg/dl)	4,0	1,8
LDH	(U/l)	942	321
Reticulocytes	(‰)	541	187
Haptoglobin	(mg/dl)	–	–

Discussion

From the course of observation made from April to August 1980 (table I), it is evident that, compared with the laboratory tests at the time of admission, an increase in erythrocytes and Hb values as well as a decline of bilirubin, LDH, and reticulocytes were achieved. At the time of release from the hospital, haptoglobin could still not be measured.

In a few cases of autoimmune hemolytic anemia that proved refractory to conventional therapy, the plasma-exchange therapy has been employed with success [5, 6]. While acute cases of other autoimmune diseases responded well to plasma exchange therapy, no continuing improvement could be recorded for chronic cases [7, 8]. The same could be reported for the case described here. Autoimmune hemolytic anemia was present in this patient 6 weeks after diagnosis; the plasma-exchange therapy was not able to effect a reduction of the erythrocytic antibody load nor any essential improvement in the hemolysis parameter. Conversely, a rise in thrombocytes occurred and thrombocytic antibodies were no longer detectable. The question remains whether this effect would have also resulted from application of plasma-exchange therapy without concurrent immunosuppression. Observations made on a patient with myasthenia gravis suggest that a synergistic effect is present [9]. We consider plasma-exchange therapy to be a sensible complement to conventional immunosuppressive therapy, especially in acute and life-threatening cases.

References

1   Evans, R. S.; Takahashi, K.; Duane, R. T.; Payne, R.; Liu, Ck.: Primary thrombocytopenic purpura and acquired hemolytic anemia: Evidence of a common etiology. Archs intern. Med. *87:* 48 (1951).

2   Mönch, H.; Breithaupt, H.; Mueller-Eckhardt, C.: Immunological studies in a case of Evans' syndrome. Blut 42: 27 (1981).
3   Mueller-Eckhardt, C.; Schulz, G.; Sauer, K. H.; Dienst, C.; Mahn, I.: Studies on the platelet radioactive anti-immunoglobulin test. J. immunol. Methods 19: 1 (1978).
4   Kabat, E. A.; Mayer, M. M.: Experimental Immunochemistry, p. 135 (C. C. Thomas Publishers, Springfield, Illinois 1961).
5   McCullough, J.; Fortuny, I. E.; Kennedy, B. J.; Edson, J. R.; Branda, R. F.; Jacob, H. S.: Rapid plasma exchange with the continuous-flow centrifuge. Transfusion 13: 94 (1973).
6   Taft, E. G.; Propp, R. P.; Sullivan, S. A.: Plasma exchange for cold agglutinin hemolytic anemia. Transfusion 17: 173 (1977).
7   Daudona, P.; Nathan, A. W.; Marshall, N. J.; Bidey, S.; Havard, C. W.: Plasmapheresis as treatment for acute fulminant endocrine exophthalmos. NHK 9: 139 (1980).
8   Roujeau, J. C.; Revuz, J.; Fabre, M.; Mannoni, P.; Tourdine, R.: Plasma exchanges in pemphigus vulgaris. NHK 9: 148 (1980).
9   Dau, P. C.; Poole, M.: Plasmapheresis in myasthenia gravis. NHK 9: 139 (1980).

Dr. med. Helga Mönch, Medizin. Universitätsklinik, Abt. Hämatologie/Onkologie, Robert-Koch-Str. 40, D-3400 Göttingen

Effect of Early Plasmapheresis and High-Dose Cyclophosphamide Therapy in Goodpasture's Syndrome

H. H. Euler[1], L. Kleine[1], H. J. Gutschmidt[2], J. D. Herrlinger[1]

[1] II. Medizinische Klinik der Universität Kiel, FRG
[2] Abteilung für Intensiv-Medizin und Dialyse des Städtischen Krankenhauses Kiel, FRG

Goodpasture's syndrome (GS) (first description [18]) is defined as a rapidly progressive injury to the basement membranes of the lungs and kidneys caused by autoantibodies (anti-glomerular basement membrane antibodies, ABM-AB) [4, 29, 30, 37, 48]. GS is distinguished from ABM-AB-positve, rapidly progressive glomerulonephritis and interstitial nephritis by its additional pulmonary manifestation [22, 30, 45]. In addition to its typical clinical picture, characterized by abruptly commencing hemoptysis and hematuria, extending to a fatal respiratory insufficiency and anuria, GS must be diagnosed on the basis of high titers of ABM-AB [48]. Certain cases of GS are known to have primarily pulmonary and only few renal manifestations [32, 39].

GS is most often observed in young men. Exogenous factors are being discussed for triggering the autoaggression [3, 48].

Case Data

A. H., 21 years old, was until his hospitalization healthy, but for the last 5 years had been addicted to drugs (primarily LSD). For 2 years he had been taking almost daily, as a drug substitute [15, 21, 26], high doses of the antitussive medication isoaminile citrate (up to 60 pearls of Peracon® = 2.4 g/day). He temporarily ceased taking isoaminile citrate, for the first time, 4 days before hospitalization when increasing dyspnea and tachycardia appeared as well as a weight gain of approximately 5 kg associated with edema. In the following days, he clearly felt better. However, as the signs of withdrawal increased, he again consumed 1.6 g of isoaminile citrate. Approximately 4 h later, the appearance of pronounced dyspnea at rest led to his admission to the hospital with the diagnosis of suspected toxic, hemorrhaging pulmonary edema.

The athletic patient was in a considerably weakened general condition. When he arrived at the intensive care unit, a pronounced dyspnea at rest, edema of the ankles and face, and cyanosis were present. Immediately after his admission, attacks of massive hemoptysis accompanied by bloody, frothy lung edema resulted in respiratory standstill. Intubation was applied to the intensely cyanotic patient and he was artificially supplied with air (p = 45 cm H_2O, PEEP = 5 cm H_2O, arterial pO_2 maximally = 65 mmHg). X-ray examination revealed a typically fluid lung (fig. 1); only peripheral areas in the upper and lower lung sections still showed a normal transparency (RR 240/140 mmHg). Urinalysis showed massive presence of erythrocytes and granulated urinary cylinders. Despite good diuresis under administration of furosemide (9200 ml in the first 48 h), the retention of substances normally eliminated in the urine increased (table I). Leukocyte count was 28.7×10^3/cmm, Quick's test = 33%; other laboratory data were in the normal range. The hemoptysis and hematuria with increasing respiratory and renal insufficiency were interpreted to indicate Goodpasture's syndrome.

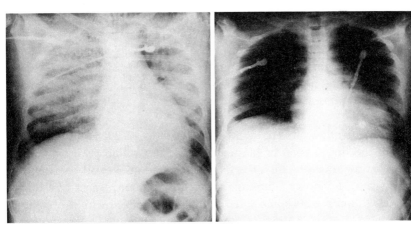

Fig. 1. Patient A. H., Goodpasture's syndrome, before first plasmapheresis.

Fig. 2. Patient A. H., G. S., 48 h after first plasmapheresis.

Table I. Patient A. H.: Survey of patient material

Day	3*	5**	8	16	180
Anti-glomerular basement membrane antibodies	+++	(+)	∅	∅	∅
C_3 (mg/dl)	21	47	88	109	105
BUN (mg/dl)	58	42	19	15	16
Creatinine (mg/dl)	2,9	1,6	1,1	0,9	0,9
pO_2 (mmHg)	39	55	83	83	–
Hematuria	++++	+++	(+)	(+)	∅

* before first plasmapheresis
** after second plasmapheresis

Proof of high titers of anti-glomerular basement membrane antibodies (indirect immunofluorescence, Prof. Vorlaender, Berlin) confirmed the diagnosis. At the same time the third component of complement was reduced, indicating thus a complement consuming AG–AB reaction (table I).

Despite positive end-expiratory pressure respiration, heparinazation and daily administration of 100 mg of prednisone, there was no improvement. On the 3rd day after admission, plasmapheresis and cytostatic treatment (immunosuppression) were begun at first without knowledge of the ABM-AB titer.

Via a femoral Seldinger catheter, 12 × 500 ml venous blood were drawn over a period of 6 h into vacuum flasks with stabilizer; these were then centrifuged at 4° C for 10 min at 750 × g. The supernatant was discarded, the sediment was resuspended with physiologic saline solution and human albumin, and then reinfused. This procedure was repeated after 48 h; a total of 6.5 l plasma was extracted from 12 l blood. In parallel 600 mg cyclophosphamide were administered i. v. (= 9 mg/kg body wt.) on days 3–6.

The patient was able to breathe without assistance 6 h after the beginning of the first session of plasmapheresis, and within 48 h his general condition improved rapidly: the facial edema and the swollen ankles disappeared, and x-rays of the lung showed only minor traces of shadows (fig. 2). Blood pressure and urine findings normalized within 1 week. A daily p. o. dose of 50 mg of prednisone was continued for another 3 weeks.

After a total of 4 weeks the patient was in a symptom-free condition and could be released. There has still been no relapse within 18 months, and the ABM-AB titer remains negative (table I).

The patient refused renal biopsy, since he was convinced that the intake of isoaminile citrate had caused the attacks. An intracutaneous test with 0.2 ml isoaminile citrate solution showed neither the local picture of an immediate nor of a late immunologic reaction.

Discussion

Until 1975 the prognosis for GS was basically unfavorable (survey: 4.32). Cause of death was terminal renal insufficiency, hemorrhagic shock due to hemoptysis, and fatal respiratory insufficiency. Therapeutic approaches included administration of corticoids [25], anticoagulation [27], and bilateral nephrectomy [5, 8, 48].

After *Lockwood et al.* [31] introduced the combination of immunosuppressive therapy with plasmapheresis, the prognosis improved. There is a total of approximately 40 case-descriptions in which this treatment has been applied. On the average, a 6-month period of treatment is described, and only rarely do deaths occur after this treatment [32]. However, about half of the patients remain dependent on dialysis [1, 12, 22–24, 32, 33, 35–37, 43], and complete remissions are still rare [29, 32, 46] (in each case lasting for at least 6 months). The remaining cases can be termed only partial remissions, since symptoms remain, e. g. renal insufficiency not requiring dialysis [6, 7, 12, 13, 19, 22, 31–33, 38, 48]. Individual cases have been reported in which hemoptysis reappears after plasmapheresis treatment is ceased [33] or else renal function rapidly deteriorates [34, 47].

With only one exception [36], all cases involved concurrent treatment with immunosuppressive agents and corticoids. The dosage scheme for cyclophosphamide was 1 to maximally 3 mg/kg/day over a period of 2–50 weeks, generally for 4 weeks. In individual cases, azathioprine was administered instead of cyclophosphamide in dosages of 1–2 mg/kg/day [1, 6, 17, 29, 37]; only rarely were both substances administered concurrently [32]. In all cases, 30–250 (generally 100) mg prednisone/day were administered in parallel for 3–50 (generally 4) weeks. The hypothetic goal of this procedure has been to prevent an excessive reactive formation of ABM-AB following the elimination of these antibodies when antigens are suspected to persist [4, 8, 22, 32, 39]. Experimental results support the assumption that a short-term high-dose cyclophosphamide therapy can functionally eliminate a stimulated clone of proliferating immunecompetent cells [20]. These findings induced us to apply higher doses of cyclophosphamide for a shorter period of time than usual.

Approximately 45% of the pathogenic IgG (rarely IgA [13]) in illnesses induced by ABM-AB circulate in the serum; the remaining AB are distributed throughout the extravascular area. To avoid a reactivation of the clinical picture of the disease via redistribution of the tissue-bound AB into the serum all authors suggest or apply repeated plasmapheresis [23, 24]. Discontinuous-flow and continuous-flow (less often) procedures are applied. Generally 3–4 l of plasma are exchanged per plasmapheresis session; less often, 1 l [22] or 2 l [7, 33, 36]. The more recent reports show a trend to exchange larger volumes: 4.5 l [46], 5 l [1, 17, 22, 37, 38]. There is considerable fluctuation in the frequency of plasmapheresis and the total number of sessions. Three plasmapheresis sessions per week predominate, applied over a period of 2–4 weeks (maximally 46 × 4 l in 12 weeks [43]).

Since 1977, the original method of plasmapheresis using centrifugation, mostly via cell separators, has been increasingly abandoned in favor of the simpler technique (if hemofiltration systems are available) of plasmapheresis via hollow-fiber membranes (Plasmaflo, Asahi PF 01) [1, 2, 16, 17, 37, 40–42]. Compared with the centrifugation method, plasmapheresis with hollow-fiber membranes is a less radical procedure. Via the membranes, the antibodies of the IgG class are filtered out by approximately 65% [2, 8, 40]; macromolecular substances, such as IgM, by 59% [41]; and fibrinogen by only about 30% [41]. Consequently immune complexes, whose role in the pathogenesis of GS has not yet been clarified [28, 39] are supposed to be filtered out by only a small percentage. A further problem of plasmapheresis with membranes can be posed by the possible development of secondary membranes with lessening filtration rates over time [1, 16]. In contrast, centrifugation plasmapheresis eliminates equally all components of plasma by approximately 85%. We favored this method.

In all the cases described, there was an initial fall of ABM-AB titers. Normally after 2–4 weeks (exception: 6 days [17]), no ABM-AB could be detected in approximately 2/3 of the cases. In the rest, ABM-AB remained detectable throughout the reported period [1, 22–24, 32, 43].

Those cases of GS in which pulmonary manifestation prevailed over renal manifestations responded faster and longer to the therapy [12, 13,

29, 33, 46]. Patients who were already anuric at the beginning of the therapy remained requiring dialysis [1, 22, 24, 32, 36, 43]. In non-anuric patients, the therapy achieved a slow improvement of renal function [6, 7, 22, 31, 33, 38]. If both strong hemoptysis and renal symptoms were observed, the therapy first led to an improvement of the respiratory situation as opposed to a slower improvement of the renal insufficiency [10, 22, 32, 33, 43]. This may be explained by a reduced binding of ABM-AB to the pulmonary antigen structures.

The most important factor for the prognosis of GS seems to be the period between the first manifestation of the disease and the beginning of therapy. Whereas the first reports dealt with a course of illness beginning several months (up to 5 years [35]) prior to therapy, the more recent works show a tendency to a shorter interval between the first attack of hemoptysis and beginning of therapy (2–6 weeks [1, 12, 22]).

The possibility of an exogenous or drug-induced etiology of GS, perhaps via hapten mechanisms, has been discussed, e. g., for D-penicillamine [28, 44], phenytoin [44], and hydrocarbons [3]. However, proof for the existence of this pathogenetic chain has not yet been found. Also, in our case only the temporal co-occurrence of isoaminile citrate intake and the appearance of clinical symptoms indicates the possibility of a causal connection.

Our experience recommends treatment of GS as early as possible – especially its pulmonary manifestations – by large-volume plasmapheresis combined with a short-term administration of high-dose cyclophosphamide.

References

1   Arnold, P.; Dieker, P.: Experiences in often repeated plasma separation by membrane in a case of Goodpasture's syndrome. Nieren- u. Hochdruckkrankht. 9: 136 (1980).
2   Asaba, H.; Löfqvist, B.; Wehle, B.; Bergström, J.: Plasma exchange with a membrane plasma filter (plasmaflo). Nieren- u. Hochdruckkrankht. 9: 136 (1980).
3   Beirne, G. J.; Brennan, T.: Anti-glomerular basement membrane antibody-mediated glomerulonephritis associated with chronic exposure to hydrocarbon solvents. Archs envir. Hlth 25: 365 (1972).
4   Benoit, F. L.; Rulon, D. B.; Theil, G. B.; Doolan, P. D.; Watten, R. H.: Goodpasture's syndrome. Am. J. Med. 37: 424 (1964).
5   Bergrem, H.; Jervell, J.; Brodwall, E. K.; Flatmark, A.; Mellbye, O.: Goodpasture's syndrome. A report of seven patients including long-term follow-up of three who received a kidney transplant. Am. J. Med. 68: 54 (1980).
6   Borberg, H.; Kindler, J.; Mahieu, B.; Sladecek, I.; Tschöpe, W.; Sieberth, H. G.; Gross, R.: Zur Behandlung des Goodpasture Syndroms. Med. Welt 29: 545 (1978).

7   Bruns, F. J.; Stachura, I.; Adler, Sh.; Segel, D. P.: Effect of early plasmapheresis and immunosuppressive therapy on natural history of anti-glomerular basement membrane glomerulonephritis. Archs intern. Med. *139:* 372 (1979).

8   Cove-Smith, J. R.; McLeod, A. A.; Blamey, R. W.; Knapp, M. S.; Reeves, W. G.; Wilson, C. B.: Transplantation, immunosuppression, and plasmapheresis in Goodpasture's syndrome. Clin. Nephrol. *9:* 126 (1978).

9   Dahlberg, P. J.; Kurtz, S. B.; Donadio, J. V., Jr.: Recurrent Goodpasture's syndrome. Mayo Clin. Proc. *53:* 533 (1978).

10 Depner, T.; Chaffin, M.; Wilson, C.; Gulyassy, P.: Plasmapheresis for severe Goodpasture's syndrome. Kidney int. *8:* 409 (1975).

11 Erickson, St. B.; Kurtz, S. B.; Donadio, J. V., Jr.; Holley, K. E.; Velosa, J.; Wilson, C. B.; Pineda, A.: Treatment of Goodpasture's syndrome by plasmapheresis and immunosuppression. Kidney int. *11:* 650 (1978).

12 Erickson, St. B.; Kurtz, S. B.; Donadio, J. V. Jr.; Holley, K. E.; Wilson, C. B.; Pineda, A. A.: Use of combined plasmapheresis and immunosuppression in the treatment of Goodpasture's syndrome. Mayo Clin. Proc. *54:* 714 (1979).

13 Espinosa-Meléndez, E.; Forbes, D. C.; Hollomby, D. J.; Katz, M. G.: Goodpasture's syndrome treated with plasmapheresis. Archs intern. Med. *140:* 542 (1980).

14 Finch, R. A.; Rutsky, E. A.; McGowan, E.; Wilson, C. B.: Treatment of Goodpasture's syndrome with immunosuppression and plasmapheresis. South Med. J. *72:* 1288 (1979).

15 Gielsdorf, W.; Holz, H.: Isoaminil als Ausweichdroge. Dt. Apotheker-Zeitung *120:* 1353 (1980).

16 Glöckner, W. M.; Sieberth, H. G.: Plasmafiltration, a new method of plasma exchange. Proc. Eur. Soc. artif. Organs *5:* 214 (1978).

17 Glöckner, W. M.; Kindler, J.; Vlaho, M.; Maerker-Alzer, G.; Mahieu, P.; Sieberth, H. G.: Antikörper-Eliminierung mittels Plasmafiltration über Hohlfasermembranen am Beispiel des Goodpasture-Syndroms. Verh. dt. Ges. inn. Med. *85:* 76 (1979).

18 Goodpasture, E. W.: The significance of certain pulmonary lesions in relation to the etiology of influenza. Am. J. med. Sci. *158:* 863 (1919).

19 Goudable, C.; Segonds, A.; Eschapasse, Y.; Ton That, H.; Durand, D.; Gassia, J. P.; Suc, J. M.: Plasma separation in a Goodpasture's syndrome associated with angeitis. Nieren- u. Hochdruckkrankht. *9:* 142 (1980).

20 Herrlinger, J. D.: Antigenspezifische Unterdrückung der Antikörperbildung sensibilisierter Tiere (Gustav Fischer Verlag, Stuttgart–New York 1979).

21 Iffland, R.: Die Verwendung von Isoaminil als Drogenersatz. Z. Rechtsmed. *72:* 124 (1973).

22 Johnson, J. P.; Whitman, W.; Briggs, W. A.: Plasmapheresis and immunosuppressive agents in antibasement membrane antibody-induced Goodpasture's syndrome. Am. J. Med. *64:* 354 (1978).

23 Kamanabroo, D.; Intorp, H. W.; Samizadeh, H.; Loew, H.: Erfolgreiche Behandlung des Goodpasture-Syndroms mit Plasmapherese in Kombination mit Cyclophosphamid und Glukokortikoiden. Verh. dt. Ges. inn. Med. *83:* 856 (1977).

24 Kamanabroo, D.; Intorp, H. W.; Loew, H.; Müller, K.: Plasma exchange in combination with cytotoxic drugs and corticosteroids in the treatment of Goodpasture's syndrome. Nieren- u. Hochdruckkrankht. *9:* 144 (1980).

25 Kopelman, R.; Hoffstein, P.; Klahr, S.: Steroid therapy in Goodpasture's syndrome. Ann. intern. Med. *5:* 734 (1975).

26 Kiehlholz, P.; Ladewig, D.: Über Drogenabhängigkeit bei Jugendlichen. Dt. Med. Wschr. *95:* 101 (1970).

27 Kincaid-Smith, P.: Coagulation and renal disease. Kidney int. *2:* 183 (1972).

28 Kirby, J. D.; Dieppe, P. A.; Huskisson, E. C.; Smith, B.: D-penicillamine and immune complex deposition. Ann. rheum. Dis. *38:* 344 (1979).
29 Lang, C. H.; Brown, D. C.; Staley, N.; Johnson, G.; Ma, King Wai; Border, W. A.; Dalmasso, A. P.: Goodpasture's syndrome treated with immunosuppression and plasma exchange. Archs intern. Med. *137:* 1076 (1977).
30 Lerner, R. A.; Glassock, R. J.; Dixon, F. J.: The role of anti-glomerular basement membrane antibody in the pathogenesis of human glomerulonephritis. J. exp. Med. *126:* 989 (1967).
31 Lockwood, C. M.; Boulton, J. M.; Lowenthal, R. M.; Simpson, I. J.; Peters, D. K.; Wilson, C. B.: Recovery from Goodpasture's syndrome after immunosuppressive treatment and plasmapheresis. Brit. med. J. *ii:* 252 (1975).
32 Lockwood, C. M.; Pearson, T. A.; Rees, A. J.; Evans, D. J.; Wilson, C. B.: Immunosuppression and plasma exchange in the treatment of Goodpasture's syndrome. Lancet *iii:* 711 (1976).
33 McKenzie, P. E.; Taylor, A. E.; Woodroffe, A. J.; Seymour, A. E.; Chan, Y.-L.; Clarkson, A. R.: Plasmapheresis in glomerulonephritis. Clin. Nephrol. *12:* 97 (1979).
34 McLeish, K. R.; Maxwell, D. R.; Luft, F. C.: Failure of plasma exchange and immunosuppression to improve renal function in Goodpasture's syndrome. Clin. Nephrol. *10:* 71 (1978).
35 Misiani, R.; Bertani, T.; Licini, R.; Remuzzi, G.; Mecca, G.: Asphyxia in Goodpasture's syndrome: Early treatment by immunosuppression and plasma exchange. Lancet *i:* 552 (1978).
36 Munk, Z. M.; Skamene, E.: Goodpasture's syndrome effects of plasmapheresis. Clin. exp. Immunol. *36:* 244 (1979).
37 Oldenbroek, C.; Bakker, P.; Krediet, R. T.; Arisz, L.: Plasma filtration in the treatment of Goodpasture's disease. Nieren- u. Hochdruckkrankht. *9:* 147 (1980).
38 Rosenblatt, S. G.; Knight, W.; Bannayan, G. A.; Wilson, C. B.; Stein, J. H.: Treatment of Goodpasture's syndrome with plasmapheresis. Am. J. Med. *66:* 689 (1979).
39 Rossen, R. D.; Hersh, E. M.; Sharp, J. T.; McCredie, K. B.; Gyorkey, F.; Suki, W. N.; Eknoyan, G.; Reisberg, M. A.: Effect of plasma exchange on circulating immune complexes and antibody formation in patients treated with cyclophosphamide and prednisone. Am. J. Med. *63:* 674 (1977).
40 Schurek, H. J.; Heyde, C. v. d.; Velte, H.; Deicher, H.; Marghescu, S.; Stolte, H.: Different application of plasma exchange. Optimal adaption of exchange procedure. Nieren- u. Hochdruckkrankht. *9:* 149 (1980).
41 Sieberth, H. G.; Glöckner, W.; Hirsch, H. H.; Borberg, H.; Mahieu, P.: Plasmaseparation mit Hilfe von Membranen – Untersuchungen am Menschen. Klin. Wschr. *58:* 551 (1980).
42 Sommerlad, K. H.; Rawer, P.; Leber, H. W.: Elimination of plasma proteins during plasma separation using either centrifugation or membrane filtration. Nieren- u. Hochdruckkrankht. *9:* 150 (1980).
43 Swainson, C. P.; Robson, J. S.; Urbaniak, S. J.; Keller, A. J.; Kay, A. B.: Treatment of Goodpasture's disease by plasma exchange and immunosuppression. Clin. exp. Immunol. *32:* 233 (1978).
44 Swainson, C. P.; Urbaniak, S. J.; Robson, J. S.: Plasma exchange in the successful treatment of drug-induced renal failure. Nieren- u. Hochdruckkrankht. *9:* 150 (1980).
45 Theofilopoulos, A. N.; Dixon, F. J.: The biology and detection of immune complexes. Adv. Immunol. *28:* 89 (1979).
46 Thieler, H.; Jung, N.; Schmidt, U.; Scholtze, P.; Liebetrau, G.; Gaerisch, F.; Wolf, O.; Schneider, W.: Günstiger Verlauf eines Falles von Goodpasture-Syndrom unter Plasmaaustausch und Immunsuppression. Dt. GesundhWes. *34:* 860 (1979).

47 Walker, R. G.; D-Apice, A. J.; Becker, G. J.; Kincaid-Smith, P.; Craswell, P. W.:
    Plasmapheresis in Goodpasture's syndrome with renal failure. Med. J. Aust. *i:* 875
    (1977).
48 Wilson, C. B.; Dixon, F. J.: Anti-glomerular basement membrane antibody-induced
    glomerulonephritis. Kidney int. *3:* 74 (1973).

Dr. H.-H. Euler, II. Med. Universitätsklinik, Metzstr. 53–55, D-2300 Kiel 1

Plasma Exchange in a Case of Wegener's Granulomatosis

B.-R. Suchy[1], R. Schley[2], K. Nogai[2], J. Bennhold[2], W. Pribilla[2]

[1] Onkologische Abteilung, Rudolf-Virchow-Krankenhaus, Berlin, FRG
[2] II. Innere Abteilung, Krankenhaus Moabit, Berlin, FRG

Plasmapheresis seems to be an interesting therapeutic approach in cases of immunological disorders [3–6]. Therefore the following case-report of Wegener's granulomatosis will be presented.

History

A 45-year-old female patient had a long-lasting infection of the upper respiratory tract which was resistant to therapy. In addition, she had migrating arthritis-like pain and an ulcer in the mucosal membrane of the nose.

At the time of admission to the hospital, her creatinine level was 12 mg% and urine volume 600 ml per 24 h. Urine sediment contained an abundance of erythrocytes and an x-ray film of the lungs revealed patchy bilateral infiltrates. During the patient's first 3 days of hospitalization, she underwent hemodialysis in three 5-h sessions. On hospital day 7, daily medication with 100 mg methyl-prednisolone was started. The patient did not respond. The creatinine level rose to 15 mg% without dialysis; the urinary volume decreased to 0–200 ml per 24 h; hematuria and pulmonal infiltrates persisted (fig. 1–3).

As a preliminary diagnosis an immunological disorder affecting the lungs and kidneys was assumed and therapeutic plasmaphereses were started.

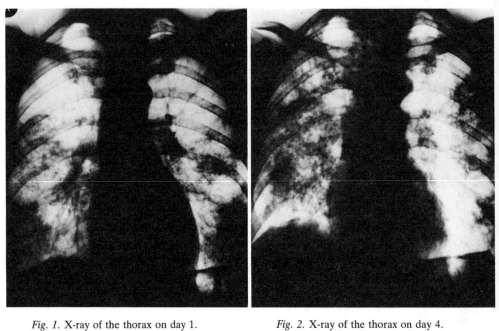

Fig. 1. X-ray of the thorax on day 1.   *Fig. 2.* X-ray of the thorax on day 4.

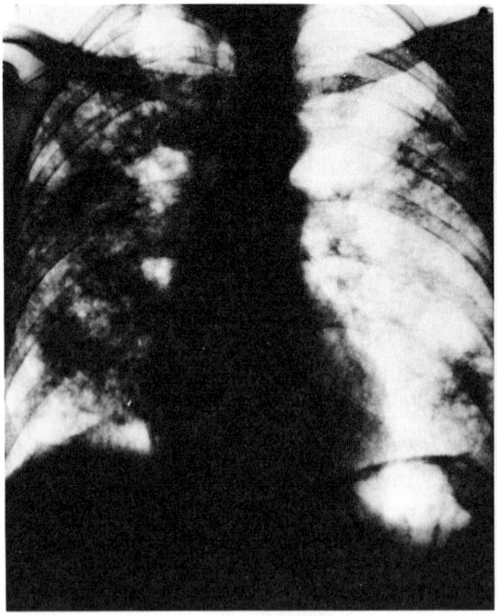

Fig. 3. Day 15, one day before plasma exchange. 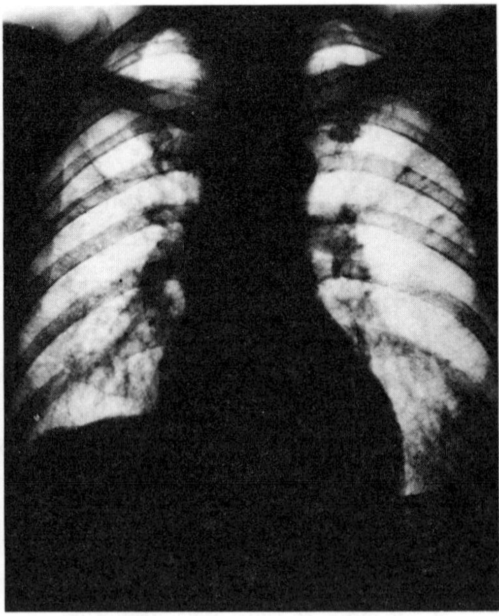   *Fig. 4.* Two days after 2nd plasma exchange.

Methods (an Aminco-Celltrifuge was used)

The inputline was connected to a Seldinger catheter in a femoral vein. Blood flow remained constant at 60 ml/min and the rotor speed was 1600 rpm. Anticoagulation was started by a bolus injection of 2000 U of heparin and 2–3 ml ACD-A/60 ml blood flow was continuously pumped into the inputline. The plasma and the buffy coat (which consisted mainly of platelets and lymphocytes) were collected separately. Replacement of the separated plasma was achieved by infusion of salt solution, human albumin 20%, fresh-frozen plasma, serum conserve (Biseko®), and 500 ml of 12-h-old whole blood. These solutions were warmed to 37° C. Finally, the buffy coat was reinfused. The patient's plasma volume was 2200 ml. During the initial plasma exchange, 2609 ml plasma was replaced by 500 ml Ringer's solution, 50 ml human albumin, 500 ml fresh-frozen plasma, 250 ml Biseko, and 500 ml blood. During the plasma exchange heart frequency and blood pressure remained constant. The patient appeared well after the treatment, which lasted 75 min.

During the second plasma exchange, we exchanged 3946 ml plasma and substituted a total volume of 3200 ml comprising 2000 ml Ringer, 200 ml human albumin, 500 ml fresh-frozen plasma, and 500 ml of 12-h-old whole blood. This time the plasma exchange lasted 85 min.

Results (Fig. 4)

Unfortunately the patient was hemodialysed 4 h after the second plasma exchange so that urine production remained unsatisfactory during the next 24 h.

On the following day, however, she produced 900 ml of urine and urine production has since then remained normal (with the exception of only 600 ml on day 23). The urine sediment contained only very few erythrocytes. The creatinine level never exceeded 10 mg% after this second plasma exchange and, when last measured, it was approximately 5–6 mg%.

An x-ray film of the chest 2 days after the second plasmapheresis and subsequent x-rays did not reveal any infiltrates.

Discussion

The histological examination of a needle biopsy of one kidney indicated accentuated extracapillary glomerulonephritis with granulomatous periglomerulitis.

This result, together with the clinical history of the patient, fitted well with a diagnosis of Wegener's granulomatosis [1, 2, 7]. Since the last diagnosis, the patient has been treated daily with 50–100 mg cyclophosphamid. She has never had to be hemodialysed for the last 2 years and has always felt healthy. We believe that, in this specific case, plasma-exchange had a positive effect.

References

1   Andersen, C.; Stavrides, A.: Case Report: Rapidly Progressive Renal Failure as the Primary Manifestation of Wegener's Granulomatosis. Am. J. med. Sci. 275: 109 (1978).
2   Baker, B.; Robinson, R.: Unusual Renal Manifestation of Wegener's Granulomatosis. Am. J. Med. 64: 883 (1978).
3   Editorial: Plasmaphereses and Severe Glomerulonephritis. Brit. med. J. i; 434 (1979).
4   Johnson, J. P.; Whitman, W.; Briggs, W. A.; Wilson, C. B.: Plasmaphereses and Immunosuppressive Agents in Antibasement Membrane Antibody – Induced Goodpasture's Syndrome. Am. J. Med. 64: 354 (1978).
5   Lockwood, C. M.; Rees, A. J.; Evans, D. J., Pearson, T. A.; Peters, D. K.; Wilson, C. B.: Immunosuppression and Plasma Exchange in the Treatment of Goodpasture's Syndrome. Lancet i: 711 (1976).
6   Lockwood, C. M.; Boulton-Jones, J. M.; Lowenthal, R. M.; Simpson, I. J.; Peters, D. K.; Wilson, C. B.: Recovery from Goodpasture's Syndrom after Immunosuppressive Treatment and Plasmapheresis. Brit. med. J. ii: 252 (1975).
7   Scully, R. E.; Galdabinin, J. J.; McNeely, B. U.: Case Records of the Massachusetts General Hospital. New. Eng. J. Med. 24: 1378 (1979).
8   Flaum, M. A.; Cuneo, R. A.; Appelbaum, F. R.; Deisseroth, A. B.; Engel, W. K.; Gralnik, H. R.: The Hemostatic Imbalance of Plasma Exchange Transfusion. Blood 54: 694 (1979).

Dr. B.-R. Suchy, Rudolf-Virchow-Krankenhaus, Onkologische Abteilung, Postfach 65 02 69, D-1000 Berlin 65

The Treatment of Malignant Lymphomas with Plasma Exchange

M. Klee, J.-H. Beyer[1], P. Schuff-Werner[1], G. A. Nagel

Zentrum für Innere Medizin, Abteilung Hämatologie/Onkologie, Universität Göttingen, FRG

[1] With the support of the Fazit Foundation

Introduction

The treatment of malignant lymphomas is based on the use of radiotherapy and cytotoxic medication. These established methods are, however, exhausted after the maximum dosage of radiation or medication has been reached, or in cases which develop, during the course of treatment, resistance to the usual dosage regimen of chemotherapy. We administered a series of plasma exchanges to patients with malignant lymphomas, after their disease continued to progress in spite of exhausting all possibilities offered by conventional therapy. In this study we were interested in determining whether such a course of plasma exchange therapy improves the patient's response to chemotherapy to which he was previously resistant.

Material and Methods

Three patients with Hodgkin's lymphoma and 2 with non-Hodgkin's lymphoma were subjected to a series of plasma exchanges. The treatment was carried out as a series of 3–4 exchange sessions within 7 days using the continuous-flow method with the blood-cell separator IBM 2997 [7]. During each session a plasma volume was exchanged which was equivalent to 4% of the patient's body weight (i. e., theoretically corresponding to 100% of the plasma) [12]. Either human albumin electrolyte solution

(HA) or fresh-frozen plasma (FFP) was used as plasma substitute solution [1, 3]. For anticoagulation, 5000–10 000 U heparin were initially administered i. v. and then 1000 U heparin i. v./h continuously during plasmapheresis. The same, previously ineffective, chemotherapy was then administered immediately after the series was finished or, at the latest, on the following day (see table I).

Table I. Results

Patient	Diagnosis	No. of plasma exchange series	Success	Side effects of plasma exchange
B. W. 49 y ♂	NHL	1	Clear progression with plasma exchange alone. Then renewed response to last ineffective chemotherapy & partial regression for about 3 weeks.	Chills during 1st and 2nd plasma exchanges
M. E. 70 y ♂	NHL	1	Progression could not be influenced	–
B. G. 34 y ♂	Hodgkin's disease	3	After 1st series, regression of B-symptoms and no change. After 2nd series, x-ray proof of progression in pulmonary foci but reduced B-symptoms. After 3rd series, x-ray proof of continued progression.	During 2nd exchange treatment of 3rd series, urticariay
L. M. 29 y ♂	Hodgkin's disease	3	After 1st series, partial remission. Regression of B-symptoms. After 2nd series, no change; few B-symptoms. After 3rd series, clear progression and pronounced B-symptoms.	–
G. M. 32 y ♂	Hodgkin's disease	3	After 1st series, regression of B-symptoms with only minimal doses of corticoid. Stabilization of disease and full functional capacity for 3 months. After 2nd series, renewed regression of B-symptoms and stationary behavior. After 3rd series, again no change.	–

Case Data

Case 1

B. W., male, 49 years old, with non-Hodgkin's lymphoma (lympho-blastic lymphoma).

This patient had been ill with non-Hodgkin's lymphoma since January 1979. He had been treated with telecobalttherapy using cobalt, then chemotherapy with two cycles of cyclophosphamide, oncovin, procar-bazine, and prednisone (COPP), and subsequently 3 cycles of combina-tion chemotherapy including bleomycin, adriamycin, cyclophosphamide, oncovin, and prednisone. After 10 months of this therapy, the disease proved resistant to further therapy. From 22 to 28 October 1979, four sessions of plasma exchange were carried out. During the first and second sessions, the patient experienced chills which we ascribed to the plasma substitution solution. After changing this solution, no side effects were observed in the third and fourth sessions. The tumor parameters of the patient were easily measurable. A clearly visible, large lymph-node mass was present in the left cervical and supraclavicular region. This showed a clearly visible growth during treatment with plasmapheresis alone. The subsequently applied chemotherapy, to which the patient had previously developed resistance, resulted in visible reduction of the tumor mass. Partial remission was the result which persisted for 3 weeks. Thereafter the disease progressed again. The repeated introduction of chemotherapy could no longer favorably influence the course of the disease, and the patient died on 7 December 1979.

Case 2

M. E., male, 70 years old, non-Hodgkin's lymphoma (immunocytic, polymorphous type).

At the time of diagnosis, the lymph nodes in the vicinity of the left groin were involved caudally down to the adductor canal and cranially into the area of the para-aortal lymph nodes. This was associated with secon-dary lymphatic edema of the lower extremity on the left side. The first two cycles of combination chemotherapy, including cyclophosphamide, onco-vin, prednisone, followed by irradiation of the suprainguinal and infring-uinal lymph nodes, were successful. However, at the end of radiation therapy, new manifestations appeared in the right cervical and retromandibular area. Thus, two cycles of chemotherapy, including adriamycin and bleomycin, were applied. Because of continued progression, treatment was changed to combination chemotherapy that included adriamycin, vinblastin, DTIC, and decortin. Progression persisted; a series of plasma exchanges was then instituted between the 9 and 16 July 1980. This series consisted of 4 sessions of plasmapheresis; chemotherapy according to the previous regimen followed. However, this attempt could also not halt the disease's progression, and the patient died on 27 August 1980.

Case 3

B. G., male, 34 years old, Hodgkin's disease IV B (mixed cellurarity).

The patient became ill February 1978 at the age of 32. During the following two years, he was administered an intensive cytostatic treatment. This included 6 cycles of the COPP regimen, 10 cycles of the ABVD regimen (adriamycin, bleomycin, vinblastin, and DTIC), and 4 cycles of platinum and VP 16-213. During the last-named therapy, the patient's disease was clearly progressive. X-rays showed the growth of tumor as well as new foci appearing in the lungs, and clinically, there was an increase in B-symptoms. The patient then received a series of plasma exchanges from 16 to 22 May 1980 and thereafter the same chemotherapy with cis-platinum and VP 16-213, which had previously proven unsuccessful. An impressive regression was observed in the B-symptoms, although the tumor manifestations remained otherwise stationary. Between the 24 and 30 June 1980 we carried out another series of plasma exchanges, using human albumin electrolyte solution as substitute for plasma. Immediately after this series was concluded, 17.5 g gammaglobulin was substituted, and a further cycle of chemotherapy with platinum and VP 16-213 was initiated the following day. A further regression of the B-symptoms was observed. Because of the increased formation of single, round foci in the lower right lobe of the lung as revealed by x-rays, a progression of the disease was suspected. From 31 Juli to 6 August 1980, we administered a third series of plasma exchanges with FFP as plasma substitute. Another cycle of chemotherapy including platinum and VP 16-213 was carried out the following day. Unfortunately thereafter the number of round pulmonary foci in both lungs clearly increased. Due to continuing progression, we refrained from further treatment with plasma exchange and chemotherapy.

Case 4

L. M., male, 28 years old, Hodgkin's disease, initially in stage IIIA, later in IVB (lymphocytic depletion).

At first a total node irradiation was carried out. Following a relapse in December 1978 and development to stage IVB, we administered 7 cycles of COPP, followed by a short maintenance therapy with leukerin. After a further relapse, 2 cycles of adriablastin, bleomycin, DTIC, and decortin, as well as a cycle of chemotherapy containing adriablastin, VP 16-213, and DTIC followed. Thereafter a chemotherapy cycle with platinum and VP 16-213 was applied. Despite these measures the disease clearly progressed so that resistance to chemotherapy had to be assumed. Plasma exchange was applied from 17 to 23 May 1980. Subsequently the combination chemotherapy with platinum and VP 16-213, which had previously proved ineffective, was administered. Clinically a clear regression in swelling of the neck lymph nodes set in, and the B-symptoms completely disappeared for approximately 14 days. Thereafter the symptoms increased again, whereas the lymph nodes accessible to palpation showed no change. Between 23 and 29 June 1980 we applied another series of plasma exchanges using human albumin electrolyte solution and administered subsequently a cycle of chemotherapy with platinum and VP 16-213. Over the next approximately 4 weeks, the tumor manifestations showed a stationary behavior and there were only minor B-symptoms. At the end of July and beginning of August the size of the palpable lymph nodes rapidly increased. Thus, between 4 and 10 August 1980, we attempted another series of plasma exchanges with subsequent chemotherapy containing platinum and VP 16-213. FFP was used as plasma substitute this time. The disease continued to progress and the B-symptoms became more pronounced. Thereafter the pulmonary situation worsened; this manifested itself clinically as spastic asthmoid bronchitis. X-rays showed new, fine-spotted pulmonary foci. The patient died 7 September 1980 due to respiratory insufficiency. The autopsy of the thorax organs, carried out 8 September 1980, revealed a coarsely nodular, in part confluent, tumorous infiltration of the pulmonary parenchyma, a form of lymphogranulomatosis histologically depleted of lymphocytes.

Case 5

G. M., male, 31 years old, Hodgkin's disease IVB (initially mixed cellurarity, later lymphocytic depletion).

At the age of 26, the patient became ill in 1974 with Hodgkin's disease. The disease was already in stage IVB at the time of diagnosis and histologically appeared to be a mixed type which later developed into lymphocytic depletion. In the course of the following years, the patient underwent 25 cycles of chemotherapy with COPP regimen, cobalt irradiation (cervical, mediastinal, and iliacal areas). Subsequently he received 4 cycles of the ABVD regimen, and afterward another irradiation of a tumor in the retrotracheal area. The patient was then first administered CCNU and VM26; vindesine and amethopterine, and finally VP 16-213, platinum, and corticosteroids followed. When the disease became progressive under this therapy, a series of plasma exchanges were administered from 15 to 17 October 1979 using FFP as plasma substitute. Subsequently the patient received the chemotherapy that had previouly proved ineffective. A regression of the B-symptoms became apparent with only minimal doses of corticoids. The disease stabilized, and for another 3 months the patient showed complete functional capacity. During this time the patient received a maintenance therapy with VP 16-213. When clinical findings again indicated progression, the patient was administered another series of plasma exchanges with subsequent VP 16-213 therapy. A stationary remission again set in with decline of the B-symptoms. Upon clinical detection of a renewed progression in May 1980, another series of plasma exchanges were applied from 31 May to 6 June 1980 using HA as substitute solution. Afterward 20 g gammaglobulin were substituted and the previous chemotherapy with VP 16-213 was added. The parameters of the tumor's course remained stationary for another 2 months. In August 1980 a local swelling of the left external ear developed with high-degree pain symptoms that proved resistant to therapy. During the following period, septic temperatures developed that were resistant to antibiotic therapy. On 18 September 1980 the patient died. An autopsy identified a fungal sepsis as cause of death. Furthermore, a large part of the identified tumor foci had been necrotically transformed and in part it had also fibrosed.

Discussion

Over the last years different reports have drawn attention to the possibility of favorably influencing the course of a tumorous illnesses with plasma exchange [8, 9]. Because of the varied pragmatic treatment approaches and different procedures of plasma exchange, a uniform assessment of the role of plasma exchange in the treatment of malignomas has not been possible until now. Thus, the following questions have had to remain open:

(1) Should the positive courses be ascribed to the cytostatic therapy applied immediately following plasma exchange?

(2) Is the effect based on the removal of the so-called blocking plasma factors or immunosuppressive factors [2, 4, 6, 10, 11, 14]?

(3) Or does the addition of unknown antineoplastic factors, present in the plasma substitute solution, play a role [5]?

As our investigations show, a new response to previously ineffective chemotherapy was observed in individual cases after treatment with plasma exchange (table II).

From this it can be concluded that plasma exchange must have caused this reversal in the course of the illness, either directly or indirectly. The following explanations are possible:

Table II. Second application of chemotherapy

Success	No. of plasma exchange series n = 11	No. of patients n = 5
Renewed response to previously ineffective therapy and partial remission (PR)	2	2
Improvement of complaints with minimal response to previously ineffective therapy and stabilization of the illness (NC)	4	3
Improvement of complaints but objectively no renewed response to previously ineffective chemotherapy and progression (P)	1	1
No renewed response to the chemotherapy and progression (P). No improvement of complaints	4	3

(1) The treatment with plasma exchange removed immunosuppressive factors [9].
(2) Plasma exchange removed substances that either blocked the cytostatic effect or else the composition of the patient's plasma was altered in such a way that more favorable pharmacokinetics resulted for the cytostatic substance.

Although our experimental approach could not clarify if or which one of the above-mentioned mechanisms was effective: whether plasma exchange alone or combined with the subsequent chemotherapy caused the reversal in the course of the disease. The fact that chemotherapy alone did not lead to a reversal justifies the conclusion that plasma exchange played an important role in achieving this effect. However, this effect was obviously only of short duration. Further investigations are required to determine the role of plasmapheresis in the therapy for malignant lymphomas.

Summary

After conventional therapy had been exhausted and the disease still progressed, 3 patients with Hodgkin's lymphomas and 2 with non-Hodgkin's lymphoma were subjected to a series of plasma exchanges. After plasma exchange, the chemotherapy that was previously ineffective was applied anew to test whether a new response could be produced.

In this way 5 patients received a total of 11 series of plasma exchanges with subsequent chemotherapy. A partial remission lasting 2–3 weeks was recorded in 2 patients. Another 2 patients showed stationary tumor behavior for 3 weeks–3 months. In 1 patient, the disease's progression could not be influenced. In 2 of the 43 applied plasma-exchange sessions, chills occurred and, in 2 others, urticaria developed.

References:

1   Beyer, J.-H.; Klee, M.; Köstering, H.; Nagel, G. A.: Coagulation studies before, during, and after repeated plasma exchanges with a 5% human albumin/saline solution in normal donors. In Sieberth (ed.), Plasma Exchange, Plasmapheresis-Plasmaseparation: Internation Symposium in Cologne, June 1980, pp. 87–92 (F. K. Schattauer Verlag, Stuttgart–New York 1980).
2   Currie, G. A.; Basham, C.: Serum-mediated inhibition of the immunological reactions

of the patient to his own tumor: A possible role for circulating antigen. Brit. J. Cancer 26: 427 (1972).

3 Farrales, F. B.; Summers, T.; Belcher, C.; Bayer, W. L.: Plasma Exchange with Plasma-Protein Fraction and Lactated Ringer's Solution Using the Continuous Flow-Cell Separator. Infusionstherapie 2: 273–277 (1975).

4 Hellström, I.; Sjögren, H. O.; Warner, G.; Hellström, K. E.: Blocking of Cell-Mediated Tumor Immunity by Sera from Patients with Growing Neoplasms. Int. J. Cancer 7: 226–237 (1971).

5 Hellström, I.; Hellström, K. E.; Sjögren, H. O.; Warner, G.: Serum Factors in Tumor-Free Patients Cancelling the Blocking of Cell-Mediated Tumor Immunity. Int. J. Cancer 8: 185–191 (1971).

6 Hersey, P.; Murray, E.; Ruygrok, S.; Edwards, A.; Milton, G. W.: Blocking Factors against Melanoma Leukocyte-Dependent Antibody: Relationship to Disease Activity in Melanoma Patients. Aust. N.Z. J. Surg. 48: 26–32 (1978).

7 Hester, J. P.; Kellogg, R. M.; Mulzet, A. P.; Kruger, V. R.; McCredie, K. B.; Freireich, E.: Principles of Blood Separation and Component Extraction in a Disposable Continuous-Flow Single-Stage Channel. Blood 54: 244–268 (1979).

8 Israel, L.; Edelstein, R.; Mannoni, P.; Radot, E.: Plasmapheresis and Immunological Control of Cancer. Lancet i: 642–643 (1976).

9 Israel, L.; Edelstein, R.; Mannoni, P.; Radot, E.; Greenspan, E. M.: Plasmapheresis in patients with disseminated cancer: Clinical results and correlation with changes in serum protein. The concept of 'non-specific blocking factors'. Cancer 40: 3146-3154 (1977).

10 Israel, L.; Edelstein, R.: In Vivo and in Vitro Studies on Nonspecific Blocking Factors of Host Origin in Cancer Patients. Israel J. med. Scis 14: 105–130 (1978).

11 Sarcione, E. J.: Hepatic synthesis and secretory release of plasma alpha-2-(acute-phase)-globulin appearing in malignancy. Cancer Res. 27: 2025 (1967).

12 Siegenthaler, W.; Würsten, D.; Siegenthaler, G.: Wasser- und Elektrolythaushalt. In Siegenthaler (ed.), Klinische Pathophysiologie, pp. 196–222 (Georg Thieme Verlag, Stuttgart 1976).

13 Sjögren, H. O.; Hellström, I.; Bansal, S. C.; Hellström, K. E.: Suggestive Evidence that the 'Blocking Antibodies' of Tumor-Bearing Individuals may be Antigen-Antibody Complexes. Proc. natn. Acad. Sci. USA 68: 1372–1375 (1971).

14 Zacharia, T. P.; Pollard, M.: Elevated levels of alpha-globulins in sera from germ-free rats with methylcholanthrene-induced tumors. J. natn. Cancer Inst. 41: 35 (1969).

Dr. M. Klee, Abt. Hämatologie/Onkologie, Medizin. Universitätsklinik, Robert-Koch-Str. 40, D–3400 Göttingen

Monitoring the Course of CEA Concentration in Tumor Patients Receiving Plasmapheresis

J. Borghardt, J.-H. Beyer[1], G. A. Nagel

Medizin. Universitätsklinik, Abt. Hämatologie/Onkologie, Göttingen, FRG

[1] With a grant from the Fazit Foundation

The following data are the preliminary results from preparatory orientation studies, which were performed prior to beginning a program on the selective elimination of tumor-associated antigens by immunoabsorption.

Ever since the first reports of the *Hellströms* and a large number of recent works continuing this line of investigation, the question has become more and more pressing about the immunopathologic significance of the so-called blocking factors in the serum of cancer patients. This was our major concern in this study [1, 2, 3].

According to current experience, immunosuppressive factors, e.g., circulating immune complexes, can unfavorably influence the course of the disease, at least in some tumors. In such cases, elimination of the immune complexes by plasma exchange or specific absorption could be equally decisive, as has already been shown in autoimmune diseases. It is also known that, for example, leukemia patients with no pathologic concentration of immune complexes at the time of diagnosis, generally respond better to chemotherapy and consequently have an increased survival rate. This evidence seems to indicate that in tumor patients, who manifest progressive tumor growth during cytostatic therapy with detectable increasing concentrations of immune complexes in the serum, it would be worthwhile to attempt to eliminate these complexes in combination with subsequent chemotherapy [4, 5].

Such a plan presupposes not only monitoring the clinical course but also proving that tumor-specific, immunosuppressing substances have actually been removed. However, definitively tumor-specific antigens or immune complexes have been ambiguously detected in the human system. Therefore a measurable monitoring of their course is currently possible only by means of established substances, so-called tumor markers, which, in certain tumors, appear in significantly elevated concentrations in the patient's serum and correlate with the progression of the disease.

In accordance with the selection of our patient material (metastasizing gastro-intestinal tumors and metastasizing carcinomas of the breast), we chose carcinoembryonal antigen (CEA) as the tumor marker and measured its serum concentration in patients treated with plasmapheresis.

The following details were to be clarified:

(1) How did the tumor-associated antigens behave during elimination by the two methods of small-volume and large-volume plasma exchange?

(2) At which intervals, after treatment, did the serum concentration of CEA increase again and were there differences between the two applied procedures?

(3) Did the lowered CEA concentration lead to an improved response to chemotherapy and thus a more favorable course of the disease?

Figure 1 shows the theoretical elimination behavior of substances in relation to the exchanged volume. Since there were no intermediary membranes in our centrifugation technique used in plasmapheresis, the sieve coefficient in the figure is zero, corresponding to the straight line R = zero. Already after exchange of the simple plasma volume, it is apparent that 60% of a substance can be eliminated. However, to approach complete removal of a substance, almost 5-fold the plasma volume must be exchanged.

The evaluable cases documented here include three patients who received the so-called small-volume plasma exchange. In this procedure, the simple plasma volume was exchanged each session on every 2nd day for a total of 4 sessions. In the case of another patient, a so-called large-volume plasma exchange was undertaken, exchanging 4-fold of the calculated plasma volume in one session.

In figure 2 the serum-CEA levels found in the three patients treated with small-volume plasmapheresis are shown before, during, and after plasma exchange. One male patient with metastasizing carcinoma of the stomach had a baseline serum-CEA concentration of 900 ng/ml; one female with metastasizing carcinoma of the breast showed a baseline serum-CEA level of 700 ng/ml; and the third patient, a female with

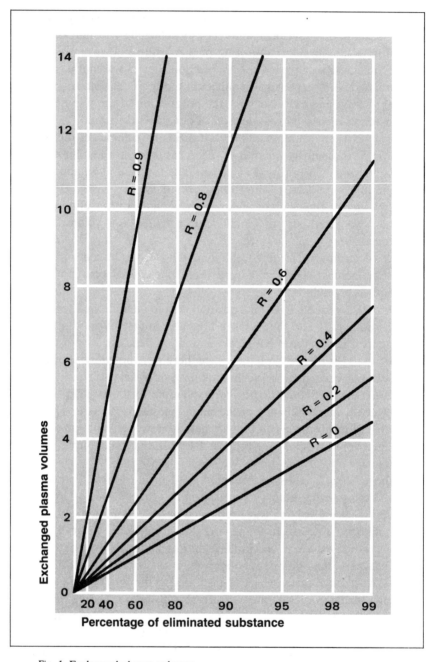

Fig. 1. Exchanged plasma volumes.

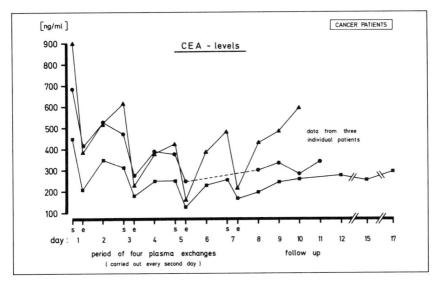

Fig. 2. Serum-CEA levels in the three patients treated with small-volume plasmapheresis.

metastasizing carcinoma of the rectum, had a baseline serum-CEA concentration of 450 ng/ml. All patients had in common the fact that they had become resistant to further treatment with cytostatic drugs. During the last cycle of chemotherapy there had been a clear tumor progression in all patients. After obtaining the consent of the patients, the only possible treatment remaining was the experimental use of plasmapheresis in combination with the cytostatic therapy that had been administered previously in each case. Figure 3 shows the serum-CEA concentration after each plasma exchange treatment. This is presented in the further course as a percentage of the baseline value. The figure shows that after the first exchange of the simple plasma volume, an average of 50% of CEA was eliminated; the theoretical elimination value was calculated in the graph in figure 1 to be 60%. Between each subsequent treatment period with plasmapheresis there is a significant elevation of the serum-CEA concentration, which, however, never reaches the baseline value. According to the data available in the meantime, which could not be taken into account in the graph, the CEA concentration stabilized to approximately 50–60% of the baseline value after conclusion of the therapy and up to 3 weeks later. Figure 4 shows the serum-CEA concentration during and after the large-volume plasma exchange mentioned above in a female patient with

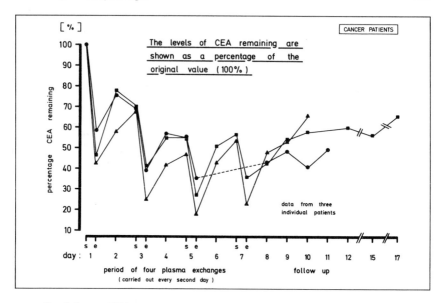

Fig. 3. Serum-CEA concentration after each plasma exchange treatment.

metastasizing carcinoma of the breast, who presented a baseline CEA concentration of 42 ng/ml. Whereas the theoretical possibility of elimination was estimated at 98% with an exchange of 4-fold plasma volume, over 90% of the serum CEA could actually be removed. In this connection, figure 5 shows the corresponding concentrations of the antigen in the separated plasma. As was seen in figure 4, monitoring the course of serum-CEA levels showed, after 3 weeks, a renewed increase of CEA concentration to approximately ⅓ of the baseline value; after 6 weeks the serum concentration was not above 50% of the baseline value.

We believe that the patient population is still too small and the period of observation, in particular, still much too short to give a conclusive answer to the question of whether or not the course of the disease was favorably influenced. However, short-term clinical improvement was observed in 3 of the 4 patients. At the present, an evaluation of the efficacy of small-volume as opposed to large-volume plasmapheresis is not yet possible. This will emerge only during the further course of the monitoring. However, without any question, sequential small-volume plasma exchange is at the present less problematic to carry out, especially as regards to rate of complications during plasmapheresis and administration of substitute solutions – it has, however, an insufficient capacity of

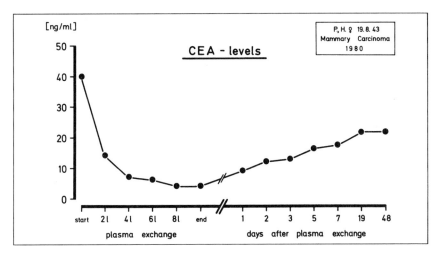

Fig. 4. Serum-CEA concentration during and after the large-volume plasma exchange.

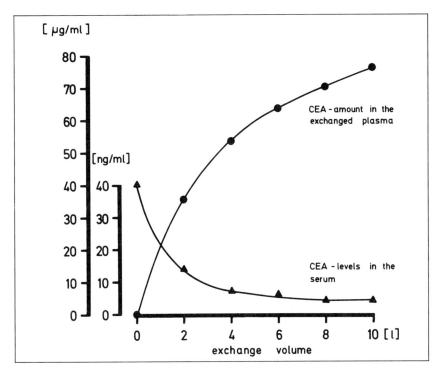

Fig. 5. CEA concentrations in the serum and CEA amount in the exchanged plasma in one patient suffering from mammary carcinoma.

elimination. Proceeding from the theoretical possibility of elimination, we are aiming at achieving a middle course: a single exchange of 2-fold plasma volume in each therapy cycle with an ideal elimination rate of 85 % for any arbitrary substance dissolved in plasma (see fig. 1). It is possible that we can still avoid substituting coagulation factors, so that human albumin would suffice as substitute solution. In this way, we could dispense with administering FFP solution (fresh-frozen plasma), which is necessary in the large-volume exchange, but which causes frequent non-tolerance reactions. With an increase of the 'clearance' by 30 % as opposed to that for the sequential small-volume exchange, the elimination rate would be only 10 % less than that of the large-volume exchange with 4-fold plasma volume. Preparations are now in progress to carry out these investigations on a larger patient population.

References

1   Hellström, I.; Hellström, K. E.: Studies on cellular immunity and its serum-mediated inhibiton in Moloney-virus-induced mouse sarcomas. Int. J. Cancer *4:* 587 (1969).
2   Hellström, K. E.; Hellström, I.: Lymphocyte-mediated cytotoxicity and blocking serum activity to tumor antigens. Adv. Immunol. *18:* 209 (1974).
3   Sjögren, H. O.; Hellström, I.; Bansal, S. C.; Hellström, K. E.: Suggestive evidence that the 'blocking antibodies' of tumor-bearing individuals may be antigen-antibody complexes. Proc. natn. Acad. Sci. USA *68:* 1372 (1971).
4   Beyer, J.-H.; Klee, M.; Kehl, A.; Krieger, G.; Bartsch, H.-H.; Borghardt, J.; Brockmeyer, J.; Kaboth, U.; Köstering, H.; Nagel, G. A.: Erste klinische Erfahrungen mit dem großvolumigen Plasmaaustausch bei Patienten mit malignen Erkrankungen. Schweiz. med. Wschr. *110:* 1447–1449 (1980).
5   Carpentier, N. A.; Lange, G. T.; Fiere, D. M.; Fournie, G. J.; Lambert, P. H.; Miescher, P. A.: Clinical relevance of circulating immune complexes in human leukemia. Association in acute leukemia of the presence of immune complexes with unfavorable prognosis. J. clin. Invest. *60:* 874 (1977).

Dr. J. Borghardt, Medizin. Universitätsklinik, Abt. Hämatologie/Onkologie, Robert-Koch-Str. 40, D–3400 Göttingen